Advance Praise for *The Bodywise Woman*

No group has done more than Melpomene to research the psychology, sociology, and physiology of active women. Now they've brought their findings together in a book that will help you feel stronger, healthier, and more energized than you ever imagined possible.

—Amby Burfoot, Executive Editor,
Runner's World Magazine

The *Bodywise Woman* is a book that no woman should be without! For the first time you will find all the answers to those questions about *exercise and you* between the covers of one book. And once you've read the evidence substantiated by research, you will be convinced that you cannot afford *not* to exercise.

—Dorothy V. Harris, Professor,
Exercise and Sports Science, Penn State

As a researcher in the area of women and sport, I was particularly impressed by the quality of information provided in *The Bodywise Woman*. The facts are corroborated with scientific research, yet presented in a very readable fashion. From chapters about menstruation and exercise to pregnancy to old age, there is something in this book for everyone who is interested in the relationship between exercise and health for women.

—Linda Bunker, Past President,
Sport Psychology Academy,
Professor, University of Virginia

THE
BODYWISE
WOMAN

Reliable Information
About Physical Activity
and Health

BY THE STAFF AND RESEARCHERS OF

THE MELPOMENE INSTITUTE
FOR
WOMEN'S HEALTH RESEARCH

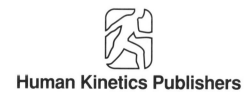

Human Kinetics Publishers

Library of Congress Cataloging-in-Publication Data

The bodywise woman / the Melpomene Institute for Women's Health
  Research.
      p. cm.
   Originally published: New York : Prentice Hall Press, c1990.
   Includes bibliographical references and index.
   ISBN 0-87322-551-1
   1. Exercise for women.   2. Physical fitness for women.   3. Women-
-Health and hygiene.   I.   Melpomene Institute for Women's Health
Research.
   [RA781.B64   1993]
   613.7'045--dc20   93-22710
                                                                    CIP

ISBN: 0-87322-551-1

The Bodywise Woman was previously published by Prentice Hall Press. Starting in 1993, *The
Bodywise Woman* is available exclusively from Human Kinetics Publishers.

Printer: Versa Press

Printed in the United States of America

10   9   8   7   6   5   4   3   2   1

Human Kinetics Publishers
P.O. Box 5076, Champaign, IL 61825-5076
1-800-747-4457

Canada: Human Kinetics Publishers, P.O. Box 2503, Windsor, ON N8Y 4S2
1-800-465-7301 (in Canada only)

Europe: Human Kinetics Publishers (Europe) Ltd., P.O. Box IW14,
Leeds LS16 6TR, England
0532-781708

Australia: Human Kinetics Publishers, P.O. Box 80, Kingswood 5062, South Australia
618-374-0433

New Zealand: Human Kinetics Publishers, P.O. Box 105-231, Auckland 1
(09) 309-2259

AUTHORS

Judy Mahle Lutter
Lynn Jaffee
Valerie Lee
Janine Benyus
Cynthia Jones
Vicki Novak Johnson
Lee Zurek

ADDITIONAL CONTRIBUTORS

Martha Stoll Albertson
Diane Brodigan
Catherine Jordan Harnack
Tina Kalambokidis
Sharon Simpson
Megan Webster

ACKNOWLEDGMENTS

Special thanks to:

Lael Berman, Janis Dees, Kay Denny, Irene Duckett-Cass, Pat Kulpa, Lowell Lutter, Arnette Nelson, Susan Olstad Peterson, Boeckmann Library at Ramsey County Medical Society/United Hospital, Beatrice (Bean) Robinson.

We also thank:

Boston Women's Health Book Collective, Vancouver Women's Health Collective, Melpomene Institute Members and Study Participants, Women's Sports Foundation, Simi Ahuja, Irene Alton, Eva Auchincloss, Julene Bartnick, Lisa Becker, Amy Birney, Ann Bruggemeyer, Linda Bunker, Margie Burchell, Ellen Butler, Marylou Carlson, William Casey, Florence Chambers, Emily Chapman Blodgett, Sharon Clapp, Jane Curry, Susan Cushman, Femmy Delyser, Jane Dick, Sally Ehlinger, Kari Goodrich, Paulette Goodrich Dow, Betty Grant, Deb Gustafson, Linda Harris, Marabai Holland, Pam Jones, Julie Jones, Lisa Kaluza, Chris Kimber, Gretchen Kreuter, Johanna Lampe, Monica Lidral, Jill Linse, Parke Lutter, Reid Lutter, Wendy Lutter, Julia Mairs, Dick Marchiafava/Ramco Sales, Edith Mucke, Deidre Pope, Lil Racette, Sue Regnier, Judy Remington, Jenny Sargent, Mary Schwind, Joan Shapiro, Pat Sharkey, Dorothy Sheppard, Mary Lee Slettehaugh, Mary Stangle, Ruth Stricker, Pam Van Zyl York, Diane Wakat, Carol Walker, Ellen Wessel, Willie Whyte.

CONTENTS

PREFACE

Women are moving like never before. We're getting stronger, playing harder, and paying more attention to what our bodies have to say. According to the latest Women's Sports Foundation survey, 62 percent of American women over age eighteen exercise regularly. Young girls are also getting involved in greater numbers. For example, participation in girls' high school track and field has increased sixfold since 1975. College track and field participation has doubled. On the recreational front, women make up more than half the participants in the eight most popular sports in the United States. Aerobic dance is enormously popular; of the 15 million people who currently take classes 95 percent are women.

What a change from when I was young! At that time, the socialization process that started with pink and blue blankets continued in earnest on the playing fields. Little boys were encouraged to participate in athletics—through Little League, school teams, and community teams—and little girls were encouraged to grow out of their "tomboy phase" and start acting like ladies. Ladies certainly couldn't look forward to a lifetime of physical activity, much less a career in sports. Even if girls were fortunate enough to get experience on sports teams, their regular physical activity usually ended with college.

I consider myself lucky to have been an exception. When I realized I couldn't fulfill my fantasies of becoming a professional baseball player, I switched to tennis and promptly fell in love with the game. It has provided a lifetime of joy and has enabled me to feel good about my body and about myself as a person.

The sensation of being "at home" with my body is something I never take for granted. Many women are separated from their bodies by a lack of opportunity for physical activity or by a lack of knowledge about how their bodies work. Today, though opportunities have certainly improved, there are still women who are ostracized or discouraged from sport because of ability, age, size, handicap, or simply a lack of truthful information about how great exercise can feel.

Providing women with truthful information about physical activity and health is what the Melpomene Institute is all about. I first learned about Melpomene at the New Agenda Conference hosted by the Women's Sports Foundation in 1983. Melpomene was involved in exciting studies that had not been attempted before—studies that looked specifically at the effects of exercise on the female body and mind. For too long, we had been jury-rigging information from studies done on male athletes, studies that didn't really fit *us*. We had no way to disprove the myths that kept many women from even trying physical activity. Melpomene broke new ground by showing how women of all ages and abilities could benefit from sport.

I have followed Melpomene's work closely in the years since, and have visited several times to help them raise funds. When Judy Mahle Lutter, Melpomene's president, told me they were planning to write a book, I was delighted. Now that I've read it, I'm even more enthusiastic. It is not only a showcase of their impressive research findings but also a well-rounded review of other research that has been done on these topics.

After reading *The Bodywise Woman*, you'll come away with more than just the latest facts. You'll have met women who are involved in the Melpomene studies. You'll have heard their voices and lived through their experience of adolescence, pregnancy, menopause, and old age. These women are not all star athletes; in fact, most of them enjoy sports on a purely recreational level. Some are weekend walkers and some are ultramarathoners, but all have questions that are likely to have occurred to you at some time or another. Their search for answers is what made this book possible.

The thing I like most about *The Bodywise Woman* is its honesty. The authors don't pretend to have the absolute final word on women's health; they are well aware that research is a journey and that today's knowledge is merely a progress report. With that in mind, they've filled this book not with ready answers but with options and with the tools you'll need to evaluate new facts as they emerge.

The authors also know that there is no one right answer for all women. They firmly believe that you are best qualified to make decisions about your own health. If you're already enjoying the benefits of physical activity, *Bodywise* can help deepen your commitment to an active lifestyle. Or, if you're just now thinking about becoming active, *Bodywise* can also be a great companion. It welcomes you back to your own body, and invites you to feel, perhaps for the first time, "at home" there.

—Billie Jean King
Melpomene Outstanding Achievement Award Winner

MEET THE MELPOMENE INSTITUTE

When you think of an institute, do you imagine a stately brick manor with white columns and manicured lawns or a high-tech laboratory filled with serious people in white coats? Either way, you'd probably be surprised to find our comfortable, sun-filled offices located in downtown St. Paul. Come upstairs and we'll introduce you to the real Melpomene Institute.

We are a network of researchers, educators, and supporters dedicated to studying the impact of physical activity on women and girls. We are based in Minnesota, but our fourteen hundred members hail from every state in the country as well as from Canada and several foreign countries. In the eight years since we began, we're proud to have become the nation's leading source of research information on the relationship between women's health and physical activity. Our eleven part-time staff members and cadre of interns and trained volunteers conduct research on topics such as osteoporosis, body image, menstrual function, sports psychology, and exercise and pregnancy. We also publish a journal, organize conferences, maintain a resource library of three thousand articles, produce videos and informational packets, give speeches across the country, and lately, we've become book authors!

Writing this book brings us full circle. In many ways, we took this project on for the same reason that we started Melpomene: We wanted to provide up-to-date, unbiased information that would help women make informed choices about their own health and lifestyle. When we started Melpomene, we could only dream about the day when there might be enough information about women and exercise to fill a book. There was plenty known about the impact of exercise on the male body, and a few studies that looked at elite women athletes on college teams. But for the most part, the average woman who stepped out of her house to run or bike or walk every morning was operating in the dark. If she had questions about why her period had stopped, or if she could still train for the marathon now that she was pregnant, she had only one place to go—her doctor. Because of the shortage of relevant research, doctors often took a cautious approach: Stop exercising, they suggested, and whatever problems you are experiencing should go away.

For many women who were just starting to feel their endorphins, this answer was not acceptable. Judy Mahle Lutter was one of those women. It was 1973, and Judy, a thirty-three-year-old mother of three, was in desperate need of some quiet time. One day when her husband Hap, a marathon runner, came trotting in from his daily run, Judy met him at the door. "It's my turn," she told him, and before he could react, she was out the door and running around the block. Before that point, Hap had been the only athlete in the house. Judy had been a chubby kid with the nickname of "Tubs," and had shied away from anything athletic. Slowly but surely, she advanced from barely being able to make it around the block to running her first 26.2-mile marathon two years later. By 1978, the year she recorded her personal best of 2:56 at the Boston Marathon, Judy was known around town as the resident expert on women and running.

She was getting calls from women who assumed she would know about everything from nutrition to sports bras to whether or not women runners could get pregnant. Judy, in fact, couldn't answer their questions with any authority, and for that matter, she couldn't locate experts or research that would provide the answers. One of the questions that kept arising concerned the loss of periods (amenorrhea) or irregular periods. Judy, who has master's degrees in educational psychology and American studies, knew of only one way to start getting answers. She and Pat Weisner, a friend who had coached woman athletes for twenty-five years, devised a brief study questionnaire. Two national running magazines agreed to carry the questionnaire, and before they knew it, they had responses from 422 women.

The most revealing information was due to a printing fluke. Judy and Pat were unable to get all the questions on one page, so they printed the last two on the back of the sheet, with a long blank below. When they invited women to use the space for comments and questions, they had no idea they would get such lengthy responses. Nearly every woman used the space, and some even stapled extra sheets to the questionnaire. Obviously, physically active women were hungry for factual information about their bodies.

Judy and another friend, medical writer Susan Cushman, devised a twelve-page second questionnaire. It sought information about women's running history, menstrual history, contraceptive methods, physical description, and running during pregnancy. They distributed it at the 1980 Boston marathon and at the Bonnie Bell all-women 10 K race in the Twin Cities. Data from the 410 respondents revealed that most women runners, contrary to popular opinion, continue to menstruate regularly. Prior to this survey, the only research on menstruation had been done on a small group of college athletes who had shown high percentages of amenorrhea (loss of periods). Because possible causes such as diet and stress were not measured, the article left the impression that vigorous exercise always leads to amenorrhea. These results made their way into the popular media, scaring many women away from exercise. The article reporting Judy and Susan's results in the *Physician and Sportmedicine* magazine was among the first to question this assumption.

The interest generated by the survey convinced Judy and Susan to form a center for research, resources, and referral in 1981. They named their new institute Melpomene (pronounced Mel-POM-uh-nee), in honor of the Greek woman who scandalized officials by running the marathon course at the 1896 Olympics, after she had been told that women could not enter the race. Although she didn't race with the men, she did finish the course in a reputable 4 hours and 30 minutes, becoming the first woman to complete an Olympic marathon.

For the first year, Judy was the only staff person, and she worked part-time on Melpomene while holding down another job. As membership grew and the research projects took on a life of their own, Judy decided to quit her job and give Melpomene her full attention. The timing was right. The running boom was drawing thousands of women who had never before exercised, aerobic dance was beginning to mushroom, and cross-country ski races were attracting record numbers of women participants. Each time the institute's work appeared on television or in the press, the phones would ring off the hook with more questions and more thank-yous from women who were grateful that a group like Melpomene finally existed.

Melpomene was, and still is, a one-of-a-kind organization. We are different from most research institutes in at least four ways. First, we are a scientific group that manages to operate outside of a medical or academic setting. While this independence frees us from certain biases, it also presents some difficulties when it comes time to seek money from traditional granting institutions. Because we are not all physicians or Ph.Ds, we lack the "union card" that would admit us to the more common funding sources. By creatively working through other channels, we have been able to build an outstanding reputation and attract high-quality sponsors and staff. Our board of directors and advisors includes nationally recognized specialists in sports medicine, gynecology, nutrition, physical education, and psychology. They are active participants, helping to design and direct our multidisciplinary studies.

Our second unique characteristic is that we have access to a population of research subjects (our members) who range from ages thirteen to eighty-three, and who run the gamut from sideline supporters who are themselves sedentary to gold medal olympians. Between the two extremes are women who are occasionally active as well as those who try to do something active every day. Some of our members compete in a sport, but most participate purely for fun. The one thing all of our members have in common is a strong belief that physical activity does have a place in a healthy lifestyle. So far, we've conducted two studies directed exclusively at our members: one in 1981–1982 and another in 1984–1985. In the first, 197 women filled out detailed questionnaires, and in the second, we heard from 420 women. Their answers provided reams of information about the lifestyles, medical histories, attitudes, and exercise patterns of active and not-so-active women. You'll be reading about some of the results throughout this book.

Our members are not the only people we examine in our research projects, however; in fact, Melpomene members usually make up less than 10 percent of our sample populations. Most of our research subjects learn about our studies from the ads we place in newspapers, the Women's Sports Foundation newsletter and magazine, and other national magazines devoted to specific sports. For each active group of participants, we also look for a comparison group of nonactive subjects. Besides our advertised inquiries, we are also fortunate to have access to populations with which our board members and advisors work. In one study, for instance, a board member who treats scoliosis patients was able to provide expertise and access so we could look at body image perceptions of girls afflicted with this condition. Other studies look at populations that have not been examined before, such as seniors, disabled athletes, chemically dependent women, toddlers, teenagers, and large women. These broad, varied sample groups distinguish our studies from those that focus only on women in collegiate or semiprofessional sports programs. Because our samples encompass larger groups of girls and women, our findings apply to a wider range of ages and abilities.

Our studies set us apart in a third way. Rather than focusing on just one physiological function affected by exercise, our research focuses on the whole woman. We use questionnaires to gather information about eating and sleeping habits, menstrual patterns, medical history, psychological well-being, attitudes toward body image, and patterns of exercise. We follow up with measurements such as body-fat testing, x-rays, psychological evaluations, and blood testing, but the strength of our results comes from what we learn about a woman's entire lifestyle.

The ongoing nature of our studies is the fourth Melpomene trademark. When a woman becomes part of a Melpomene study, she stays part of that study for years and years. Every six months or so, we send her a new questionnaire and add her new information to the data bank. The child we study as a preschooler can expect to be with us when she's eighty. Hopefully, if she has children, they too will be part of our data bank. By following the same women through childhood, adolescence, pregnancy, menopause, and aging, we believe we'll be able to provide information that is both broader in scope and more in-depth than what is now available.

Some of our more important studies include the following:

Exercise and pregnancy. Beginning in 1981, this study took place in three phases. The first phase described the natural history of running during pregnancy for 195 physically fit women. For the second study, begun in 1983, 188 women filled out a series of questionnaires on their health and exercise history, course of their pregnancy each trimester, and experiences during labor and delivery. Follow-up surveys were sent at two and six months postpartum to monitor the health and development of the child. Other phases of the study looked at the nutritional patterns of physically active pregnant and breast-feeding women, and at the socialization of their children into sports. Among the other subjects explored in data analysis were fertility and postpartum depression of physically active women. The study was completed in 1986.

Osteoporosis. The Melpomene osteoporosis study, begun in 1982, was designed to answer questions about the relationship between long-term physical activity and bone mass fluctuations. The study provided information about the activity level, diet, heredity, hormones, bone density, health attitudes, personality characteristics, perceptions of health, body image, and other lifestyle characteristics of 111 women ages forty-six to eighty. Data were collected using the following methods: questionnaires, body density scans, diet histories, activity logs, and personal interviews. The physical activity level of the women in the study ranges from sedentary to very active. The study is ongoing.

Amenorrhea. In 1983, Melpomene began a study to document physical activity levels, eating patterns, diets, hormonal levels, bone densities, and body fat percentages of amenorrheic women and regularly menstruating women who were physically active. The study was completed in 1987.

Children's socialization study. This study was begun in 1986 to determine the factors that motivate children to become and/or stay active. Using responses from questionnaires, this study documents the physical activity patterns of children and mothers as well as the various behavioral, social, and institutional influences that may be critical to children's participation in exercise and sports. The study is ongoing.

In addition to our ongoing studies, Melpomene initiates an average of two new studies a year. We report our findings in our quarterly journal, as well as in other periodicals, books, and texts. Some of the new studies we are currently working on include the following.

Physical activity and chemical dependency. This study explores the role of physical activity for women who are recovering from chemical dependency. Our primary goal is to determine whether exercise is an important component in women's chemical dependency recovery and what effect exercise has on women who are physically active throughout recovery.

Disabled women, body image and physical activity. A pilot study, which explored the importance of physical activity and body image for disabled women, was completed in 1988. Results indicated that disabled women believed physical activity enhanced body image and provided significant psychological benefits. They cited the lack of role models, adaptive equipment, and adaptive programs as barriers. Additional research will focus on some of these concerns.

Infertility in physically active women. This study seeks to determine whether any of the various exercise factors, such as type of sport and intensity or duration of activity, has an impact on a woman's ability to become pregnant. A questionnaire addressing fertility questions, physical activity patterns, and physical characteristics such as height and weight is being distributed to women who are patients at local infertility clinics and women who are clients at local adoption agencies. Results of this study will be available in mid-1990.

Eating disorders and college athletes. This study evaluated eating behaviors and attitudes of 229 female collegiate athletes, ages eighteen to twenty-three. Participants were asked to describe their level and type of activity, body size, and weight control methods. The Eating Attitudes Test (EAT 26), a standardized screening test for eating disorder tendencies, was included in the questionnaire.

Just as important these days is our role as a clearinghouse for information on women and physical activity that is beginning to make its way into the literature and the press. We are still the only organization in the country that is specifically seeking out, organizing, and disseminating this information. We review scores of journals, newsletters, and abstracts to keep our pulse on current research of interest to physically active women. Our library of three thousand research articles is computerized for fast access. Students, educators, speakers, coaches, and individuals like yourself use our library to explore a topic in-depth or to answer a specific question. We make some of these articles available in reprint form in our informational packets on various subjects such as body image, osteoporosis, and nutrition. To get our messages to the general public, we send out nine or more press releases each year, and make numerous personal appearances on TV, radio, and lecture circuits.

As another way to disseminate and exchange information, we host two major conferences a year for doctors, other health professionals, educators, coaches, and lay people. Recent conferences on body image, maternal health and fitness, and fitness for larger women have attracted national audiences of two hundred to three hundred participants. Throughout the year, Melpomene staff members are also called to do presentations and seminars on our research for professional and lay groups. Interestingly, our conference work seems to prompt commercial healthcare organizations to develop similar educational programs. Here in Minnesota, hospitals and clinics have followed our lead and are offering classes on menopause, exercise and pregnancy, and body image.

The role of "seed-planter" has become an increasingly important one for us. Since we ourselves cannot tackle all the research questions or reach all the audiences, we have tried to ask questions and raise issues that other organizations can pursue. When we began, we were the only group that was doing research on healthcare concerns of physically active women; today we are pleased to report that new research studies are being undertaken every day. This book is an attempt to compile what's known about these topics, combining both our research and the research of others. Even as this book goes to press, there will be new findings that we won't be able to include. Instead of giving you pat answers, therefore, we've tried to give you the tools to evaluate new information as you receive it. Thus, what you learn here need not become obsolete.

Now that we've told you something about ourselves, we'd like to learn more about you. We've found that while lab tests and statistics can produce certain kinds of knowledge, our most valuable findings still come from the experiences of other women. You'll notice that checklists and exercises appear throughout the book. We invite you to photocopy these pages and send us your responses and comments. If you do, you'll be joining the thousands of women who have helped inform us, and your shared experience will help us to provide information for others.

We're thrilled to be able to pass this knowledge on to you in book form. The writing process helped us to think through some of our own assumptions and beliefs and prompted lively discussions. The deeper we dug into the topics, the more we uncovered. We met a host of new resource people and came away with a list of exciting ideas for new conferences, new research topics, and new articles for the *Melpomene Journal*. To keep our learning curve climbing, we'd like to try to answer any questions you may have after reading *The Bodywise Woman*. We also hope you'll let us know what you found particularly useful, as well as what you'd like to see changed or added in the next edition. In the meantime, a good way to keep in touch with our latest developments is to become a member by writing the Melpomene Institute at 1010 University, St. Paul, MN 55104. Our phome number is (612) 642–1951. Better yet, next time you're in the heartland, why not come upstairs and meet our "institute" in person!

—The Staff and Researchers of the Melpomene Institute
for Women's Health Research

O N E

SHOULD "LADIES" BE ACTIVE?

A Historical Look at Expert Opinions

Our mothers are amazed. We're winning racquetball tournaments, running marathons, swimming miles before work, and climbing mountains with our bikes. We're exercising in larger numbers than any other generation of women. Finally, our time has come to share in the joys and exhilaration of excelling, achieving, and transforming our self-image through sport. Now that we know how good it feels to be active, we can't help but wonder, What took us so long?

The acceptance of women in sport has not followed a steady, uphill course throughout history. Instead, it has gone through many peaks and valleys—times when female sports figures were popular heroines and times when athletic women were condemned as unfit mothers. When you start to investigate what was going on in the world during those times, you see a curious "shadow" phenomenon around women and sports. It seems that a shift in society's priorities always comes just before or behind the major movements in women's sports. Women have either been welcomed or barred from sports depending on what society needed or wanted them to be at the time. When a healthy "Rosie the Riveter" was needed during World War II, for instance, exercise was elevated to the patriotic. Then, when men returned and wanted women back at home, a rash of articles about the "dangers" of exercise appeared. Acceptance of athletic women, it seems, comes and goes depending on what kind of woman society favors at the time.

The media and the medical profession have long worked hand-in-hand to shape opinions and carry out popular agendas. Medical authorities are still called to the witness stand to either hail the benefits of physical activity, or to issue grave warnings against sport for women.

For years, misinformation kept women in bed during their periods and made them feel guilty about exercising for fear of what it would do to their reproductive organs. At Melpomene, we're strongly committed to providing women with truthful information about the effects of exercise on their bodies. But first, there are decades of myths to be dispelled. To understand how these myths began, it helps to turn back the pages of time and look at the "shadow" trends that dictated acceptance or resistance to women in sport.

CORSETS AND CLASSISM—THE VICTORIAN ERA

The nineteenth century was a period of paradox in terms of women and their bodies. Immigrants from Europe were reaching our eastern shores in droves, while at the western edge of the nation pioneer women were hacking homesteads out of the raw wilderness. For these women, the question of what to do with leisure time was moot: Survival was a full-time pursuit, and women were run ragged with fourteen-hour-a-day industrial jobs, or with chopping wood, hauling water, growing crops, herding livestock, tending to children, and building homes. Enslaved black women survived and persisted in spite of the intense physical labor demanded of them. For each of these groups, physical strength and endurance was a valued commodity and posed no challenge to a woman's femininity or fertility. On the contrary, the working class woman *depended* on her body for survival.

At the same time, middle-class and upper-class urban women were striving to appear as physically weak and helpless as they could in order to achieve "true womanhood." The "true woman," according to Victorian ideals, was passive, frail, delicate, ethereal, and soft. She was elevated onto a moral pedestal and was the keeper of her husband's last refuge—a calm, peaceful household where he could come home and forget the struggles of the outside world. To maintain her purity, the Victorian woman was urged to stay indoors, safe from the world's evils. Of course, for women in the real world who operated machines, worked in the fields, hand-washed clothing, and toiled over great kitchen stoves, this ideal was beyond reach. The only women who could actually attain this pedestal (although all were taught to aspire to it) were those of the middle and upper classes.

One of the primary functions of the Victorian "lady" was to show that her husband had really arrived at the top. If she was pale from a life indoors, it meant that she didn't have to work for a living. If she had no muscles from scrubbing floors, it meant that her husband could afford servants. The "true" woman's weak, sheltered body was actually a status symbol, separating the white gentility from the "coarse," robust lower class that served them.

Because a woman could only belong to this leisure class by attaching herself to a man, it was imperative that the Victorian woman be attractive at all times. She cultivated a white pallor with the fervor that some modern women reserve for tanning, and with the help of corsets, she achieved the illusion of having a delicate, tiny waist. No matter what size she was originally, a woman could use the wire or whalebone garment to reduce her waist by two to eight inches. Some women even had ribs removed so they could cinch themselves tighter. This abdominal equivalent of Chinese foot binding exerted an average of twenty-one pounds of pressure on internal organs, restricting circulation and displacing the liver, spleen, intestines, and bladder. If you also consider that the well-dressed woman sported up to thirty-seven pounds of street clothing in the winter (nineteen pounds of which was suspended from her waist), you can begin to understand why she fainted so often!

Ironically, the dress of the day hindered one of the primary "functions" of the Victorian lady—motherhood. Many miscarriages were caused by tightly laced corsets, and in extreme cases, a woman's uterus could actually collapse and be forced through her vagina. Because of the prevailing beliefs in medicine, a reproductive failure was the worst thing that could happen to a woman.

A WOMAN IS HER UTERUS

A large part of the Victorian woman's mystery was what lay beneath the yards of petticoats; her ability to give birth was what made her a creature composed of "finer clay" than her husband. The reproductive organs were therefore central to a woman's entire being, and the medical community believed that all sicknesses, from headaches to heart conditions to insanity, could be traced to her uterus or her ovaries. In 1849, Dr. Hollick wrote:

> The uterus, it must be remembered, is the controlling organ in the female body, being the most excitable of all, and so is ultimately connected, by the ramifications of its numerous nerves, with every other part (Ehrenreich and English 1978, 108).

Dr. M. E. Dirix concurred in 1869:

> Thus women are treated for diseases of the stomach, liver, kidneys, heart, lungs, etc.; yet, in most instances, these diseases will be found on due investigation, to be, in reality, no diseases at all, but merely the sympathetic reactions or the symptoms of one disease, namely, a disease of the womb (ibid., 110).

Perhaps because they knew so little about healthy reproductive functioning, the doctors of that time assumed that the female system was "inherently pathological," and that a woman's natural state was to be sick. Menstruation, for instance, was seen as a serious threat throughout life. According to Dr. Englemann, president of the American Gynecological Society, in 1900:

> Many a young life is battered and forever crippled on the breakers of puberty; if it crosses these unharmed and is not dashed to pieces on the rock of childbirth, it may still ground on the ever-recurring shallows of menstruation, and lastly upon the final bar of the menopause ere protection is found on the unruffled waters of the harbor beyond reach of sexual storms (ibid., 99).

According to the "experts," only a man of medicine could help a woman navigate through the dangerous waters of her life. Thus, the household doctor was an indispensable figure in upper-class families, and he was paid handsomely to "manage" the woman's many illnesses. Women were taught to trust their doctor's every word. When it came to recreational activities, the doctor's orders were to get outside, enjoy the fresh air, socialize with others of one's class, but avoid breaking into an indelicate sweat. Genteel sports of archery, croquet, bowling, tennis, and golf were the primary activities, and were usually associated with the opportunity to have respectable social encounters. Swimming was also purported to be therapeutic, but only if performed in concordance with Victorian mores of modesty and propriety.

Because the Victorians believed that the human body was indecent, both men's and women's fashions were designed to keep the maximum amount of skin covered. Of course, this idea made swimming on a public beach difficult. After struggling with how to allow women to swim and yet not bare their skin, society came up with a compromise that was more like bathing than what we think of as swimming. A woman would enter a wooden box on the beach and change into a full-length dress that was somewhat more comfortable, but certainly not more revealing. The wooden box would then be rolled into the water, where, beyond the eyes of the public, she could emerge and dunk herself. The impracticality of this arrangement was obvious to one male swimming instructor who wrote in 1903:

> Just to satisfy myself on this point of costume, I once wore a close approximation of the usual suit for women. Not until then did I rightly understand what a serious matter a few feet of superfluous cloth might become in water. The suit was amply large, yet pounds of apparently dead weight seemed to be pulling me in every direction. In that gear a swim of one hundred yards was as serious a task as a mile in my own suit. After that experience, I no longer wondered why so few women really swim well, but rather that they are able to swim at all (Howell 1982, 180).

Although more doctors were beginning to counsel women to exercise, they all agreed that activity had to cease during the "sexual storms" of a woman's menstrual period. In 1872, Dr. W. C. Taylor gave a warning that was typical of many of the popular books of the time:

> We cannot too emphatically urge the importance of regarding these monthly returns as periods of ill health, as days when the ordinary occupations are to be suspended or modified . . . Long walks, dancing, shopping, riding and parties should be avoided at this time of month

invariably and under all circumstances . . ." (Ehrenreich and English 1978, 100).

When it came to pregnancy, the warnings were particularly loud. A woman was considered "indisposed" for the entire nine months before the birth of her child and after the delivery she was advised to "recuperate" by laying in bed for many more months. These prescriptions did not seem to apply to working-class women, however. Employers gave no time off for pregnancy or recovery from childbirth, much less for painful menstrual periods. No matter how sick she was, a woman risked losing her job if she missed one day of work. The old belief that the underclasses were somehow biologically different came in handy. As Barbara Ehrenreich and Deirdre English note in their book *For Her Own Good:*

> *Someone* had to be well enough to do the work, though, and working-class women, Dr. Warner [a popular medical authority writing in 1874] noted with relief, were *not* invalids: "The African negress, who toils beside her husband in the fields of the south, and Bridget, who washes, and scrubs and toils in our homes at the north, enjoy for the most part good health, with comparative immunity from uterine disease" (ibid., 103).

"BRAIN FEVER THREATENS WOMANHOOD"

The absurdity of these contradictions was becoming obvious to many women who, as the century wore on, were growing restless in their daybeds. The suffrage movement was gaining momentum, and more and more middle-class women were seeking ways to improve themselves. They enrolled in women's colleges like Smith (opened in 1875), Wellesley (1875), Bryn Mawr (1885), and Mills (1885), and even fought to enter the all-male bastions such as Cornell and Harvard.

Higher education for women was viewed as a great experiment. Many believed that the stresses of study and life away from doctor's supervision would prove too much for the frail female composition. As Dr. Edward H. Clarke said in his frightening tract called "Sex in Education, or a Fair Chance for the Girls," the female system is not able to do two things well at once. He subscribed to a popular belief that the body was like a miniature economy, and that various parts of the body were competing for a limited pool of resources. When a woman studied, he explained, blood would be diverted to her brain, robbing essential organs of a precious life force. The organ that was in direct competition with the brain, of course, was the uterus. Clarke's book, which was so popular it had to be reprinted seventeen times, warned that higher education would cause a woman's uterus to atrophy.

To prevent this catastrophe, the founding fathers of these colleges instituted a program of physical culture that would strengthen the women to help them endure the stresses of college life. Of course, this physical culture had to be of a moderate nature, because too much physical excitement could certainly produce a nervous condition, hysteria, or even worse, a disruption of menstrual periods. The focus of the activities was on fresh air, cooperation, hygiene, and posture. Walking was most strongly encouraged as training for wifely duties such as washing, cleaning, and gardening. Other college sports included golf, tennis, croquet, archery, gymnastics, rowing, and swimming/bathing.

Women physical educators were hired to guide these activities and ensure that women did not overexert themselves or risk possible disfigurement through too much bodily contact. A Vassar College representative related that students were "positively forbidden to take gymnastics at all during the first two days of their period. They are also forbidden to ride horseback then; and, moreover, are strongly advised not to dance, nor run up and down stairs, nor do anything that gives sudden and successive . . . shocks to the trunk." Endurance sports such as track and field were discouraged because they would produce more "physical straining than physical training." Basketball was modified to minimize the possible danger of contact. The court was divided into thirds, and players (six to a team) had to stay in their third. The number of dribbles were limited and the rules penalized even accidental brushes.

GUARDIANS OF FEMININITY—PHYSICAL EDUCATORS AND THE ANTICOMPETITION MOVEMENT

Safeguarding the health of their students was only one aspect of the physical educators' job. They believed that their higher calling was to safeguard the feminine, moral nature of their students, and to keep them from falling prey to the "treacheries of competition" that "sullied" men's sports. They believed that competition bred aggressiveness and encouraged individual excellence, both of which were out of step with woman's "inborn sense of modesty and innocence." Once an athlete was singled out as a star, they argued, she would be vulnerable to commercial exploitation: People might offer her scholarships or pay to see her perform. Publicity would also violate the ideal that a woman should be unobtrusive. As one physical educator of the time noted, "The development of aggressive characteristics . . . added nothing to charm and usefulness, and were not in harmony with the best traditions of the sex." The aesthetic appeal of sports was important: We should worry about looking pretty rather than winning.

By deemphasizing individual excellence, the physical educators truly believed they were performing a service and providing "the greatest good for the greatest number." They also felt that women, who were believed to be morally superior to men, must uphold the feminine ideal. Unfortunately, women's loyalty to an antiquated, and in many ways harmful, ideal blinded them to the realities of the quickly changing world. As unbelievable as it seems, college women fought strongly to exclude women from the Olympics from 1896 to 1932. Thanks to events occurring in the larger world outside of college campuses, they found themselves fighting a rising tide of support for women in sports.

SUFFRAGETTES, BICYCLES, AND THE GOLDEN AGE OF WOMEN'S SPORTS

Despite the objections of some social commentators and medical authorities, sports were about to break out of the country clubs and college campuses and become available to all women. A number of factors contributed to the softening of society's taboos against women's sports. The suffrage movement was going strong, more women were entering the world of work, and a few glamorous sportswomen were starting to achieve fame. Slowly but surely, the spell of the Victorian ideal was starting to lose its power.

The invention of the bicycle broke the last thin barrier separating the masses from physical activity. A craze swept the country, and by 1896 there were an estimated 4 million riders using their bikes for transportation as well as for exercise. There was even a professional women's biking team. The relaxation of fashion standards was perhaps one of the most revolutionary effects of the bicycle's arrival. The skirts that women had been confined to for decades were no longer practical. Bloomers, which had been invented and considered outrageous fifty years before, finally became acceptable garb not only on the bike but in many public places. As always, a few dissenting voices tried to stem the tide of this new fad. Card-carrying puritans insisted that bicycle riding would induce sexual sensations, driving virtuous women to prostitution. Others sang the old song about bike seats being harmful to women's reproductive organs. This time, women didn't listen; they abandoned their petticoats, took to their bikes, and continued to have healthy babies.

With the coming of World War I, more women went to work in factories to support the war effort. Here, they were introduced to recreation and sports teams organized by their employers (the medical community had suggested exercise as an antidote to the long hours and poor working conditions in most factories). While the best facilities and the greatest number of teams were for men, some companies had very active women's programs. For the first time, the nation was introduced to athletes from the working class. Mildred "Babe" Didrickson, who went on to win medals in the 1932 Olympics, came out of this tradition.

Games such as basketball were popular, but the rules were changed to make distances shorter and activity less strenuous in order to "protect the femininity of women." In 1912, Dr. Dudley Allen Sargent was quoted as saying it was fine for women to be athletes, but performing "men's athletics" made women more masculine. Albert Spalding, whose name has become synonymous with sporting equipment, was also in favor of women competing in sports, as long as they didn't invade some sacred male domains. The national pastime, for instance, was to be off-limits to women. In 1911, he said:

> Neither our wives our daughters, nor our sweethearts may play Base Ball on the field. They may play Cricket, but seldom do; they may play Lawn Tennis and win championships; they may play Basket Ball, and achieve laurels; they may play Golf, and receive trophies; but Base Ball is too strenuous for womankind, except as she may take part in the grandstand (Howell 1982, 186).

What Spalding didn't realize was that American women were not paying as much attention to the "do not enter" signs posted by men. The Roaring Twenties was a decade of relaxed standards, prosperity, mobility, and a new autonomy for women. Winning the right to vote triggered a social release and made women feel as if their lives were changing. The number of women in the labor force was up 26 percent, and many were living away from home for the first time in order to be close to work. This large, new pool of women had the money and leisure time to engage in a whole host of new sports: volleyball, softball, field hockey, bowling, lacrosse, polo, fencing, swimming, skating, diving, and even sailboat racing and flying. Participants were no longer just from the upper classes, although there was some division by class depending on how expensive activities were. Industrial teams continued to be popular, and the opportunities multiplied when municipal recreation departments and agencies such as the YWCA opened their doors to women.

The period from the 1920s to the beginning of World War II has been called the Golden Age of Women's Sports. It was during this time that many sportswomen began to be nationally applauded for their prowess. Glenna Collett, the first woman to break 80 in a round of golf, won her first of six amateur championships in 1922 at the age of nineteen. In 1926, Gertrude Ederle became the first woman to swim across the English Channel, breaking the male world record by two hours. Helen Wills, known as "Little Miss Poker Face," dominated the tennis scene for most of the 1920s and into the 1930s. She won seven U.S. singles titles at Forest Hills, eight Wimbledon titles, and a gold medal at the 1928 Paris Olympics.

A GENERATION OF PLAYDAYS

Meanwhile, as women's sports were simply exploding in the world at large, female physical educators were still trying to keep women out of competitive activity. They felt more strongly than ever that women should not follow the men's pattern of intercollegiate competition. Commercialization, they feared, was like a "malignant growth which would eat at the soul of sports." In 1923, the newly formed Woman's Division of the National Amateur Athletic Federation passed a platform that shrunk what little opportunities there were for women to compete against their counterparts at other colleges. The physical educators cited "men coaches, unchaperoned travel arrangements, questionable uniforms, and the inappropriate use of women in sport advertising" as the reasons for curtailing intercollegiate competition.

In its place, they instituted a generation of play days. The idea of a play day was to bring together women from a number of schools for a day of sports activities ranging from basketball, volleyball, field hockey, and swimming to hopscotch, dodge ball, relays, and folk dancing. Individual schools would not compete against each other, but rather, each team would be composed of women from various schools. This way, supposedly, they would get to know one another, but the competitive feelings that build up in an established team would not have a chance to form. Frequent breaks for juice and cookies prevented the players from overexerting themselves and gave them time to socialize. According to the University of California Women's Athletic Association, the play days allowed women to "carry away a feeling of group loyalty and unmarred fellowship," which was more important than excelling as an individual.

Not everyone was enamored with the system, however. Eleanor Methany, an outspoken physical educator brought up during the era of play days, reflected on the stigma attached to the concept of winning:

> We had fun at those play days, and we enjoyed the tea and the sociability—but the better players among us felt frustrated by the lack of meaningful team play. These play days did little to satisfy our desire for all-out competition with worthy and honored opponents (ibid., 255).

Both the Committee on Women's Athletics and the Women's Division of the National Amateur Athletic Federation continued to support such events and to oppose programs such as the Olympic games, which they considered improper. They approved of athletics "motivated by joy and love of play, not play for the purpose of making a record or beating an opponent." Although both of these groups resisted efforts to send women to the Olympics in 1928, and again, in 1932, they were thankfully unsuccessful. By that time, women had already begun to make inroads into sporting history.

THE DEPRESSION BURSTS THE BUBBLE

The women's sports movement suffered a setback with the rest of the country when the Depression hit in the thirties. Suddenly, it was seen as unpatriotic to take a man's place in a job. Fewer women worked, went to college, or could afford to live away from home. With their freedom compromised, and the nation becoming somewhat more conservative, the freewheeling days of autonomy were over. Again, scientific evidence appeared to help escort women back to their traditional roles as homemaker and mother. In 1936, an article appearing in the prestigious *Scientific American* warned that "feminine muscular development interferes with motherhood" (ibid., 256).

Questions about athletes' femininity were also make the rounds. People could not understand women like Mildred "Babe" Didrickson, whose physical capabilities appeared to match those of a man. The gossip about the "Babe" was vicious, and even lacy clothes and a marriage did little to quell the rumors. In 1936, Lewis Terman wrote a book entitled *Sex and Personality*, in which he presented a scale that would presumably enable clinicians to determine how feminine or masculine their clients were. Curiously, he chose a scoring system that assigned negative numbers to feminine traits and positive numbers to masculine traits. Therefore, the average woman might have a score in the negative fifties, whereas an average male might score in the plus fifties. Terman found that "highly intelligent, athletic women" had scores closer to the male range than any other group of women, and scored more "masculine" than male artists. The information fed right into the hands of those who wanted to believe that sportswomen were unnatural and/or that sports participation would make a woman more masculine.

The medical misinformation and the psychological scare tactics seemed to be working. Fewer new women were joining sports leagues, and the new gymnasiums built through federal post-Depression programs were rarely filled with the joyous noise of women recreating.

EXERCISE BECOMES PATRIOTIC AGAIN—THE WORLD WAR II ERA

This time-out didn't last for long. America's entry into the Second World War was a powerful "shadow" trend that once again changed society's attitude toward women. With millions of men in Europe, factories were desperate for workers to meet the escalating demands for supplies. Suddenly, it became not only acceptable for women to work but downright patriotic.

Four million women entered the labor force between 1940 and 1942, and they shattered the assumptions of what women could do mentally and physically. Women were drafting, driving trucks, riveting steel, and building battleships. Even in the military, wartime urgency was pushing women through doors that had never been open before. Women filled many noncombative positions in Europe, again to free males for fighting. For the first time, images of strong, able-bodied women were displayed as positive examples. It was quite a departure from the fixation on weak, passive, obedient housewives of a generation before!

One of the most unique results of men's absence in this country was the formation of an all-women's professional baseball league. Phillip Wrigley, owner of the Chicago Cubs, decided to see if women athletes could fill a stadium and thus fill the vacuum left by the break in men's pro ball. His gamble paid off, and the league was tremendously popular. The players were chosen for a combination of their baseball skill and feminine characteristics. The hems of their uniforms could be no more than six inches above the knee, which, when you think about it, was quite a measure of progress from the days when field hockey dresses could be only six inches from the ground! The league managed to last for twelve years, when it finally lost out to the return of the men's game, TV, and strong social pressure for women to once again return to home and hearth.

When the men came back from the war, they wanted life to be as it once had been. Although a vast majority of women wanted to keep working, many relinquished their jobs and retreated into their husband's shadow. Once again, there was plenty of expert advice encouraging the new wife and mother to stand behind her man and be available for her family. Working with her body or pursuing physical activities somehow didn't fit into the updated profile of what a family woman should be.

And, predictably, the emphasis was on protecting her most valued assets: her reproductive organs and her femininity.

Shortly after World War II, the Amateur Athletic Union (AAU) conducted a study of the effects of athletic competition on girls and women. Using a single quote from a female doctor as evidence, the organization concluded that competition during a woman's period might have a harmful effect on a woman's capacity for "being a normal mother." Even as late as the 1950s, the play day was still the most popular form of competition on most college campuses. The opportunities for sporting challenges that women had enjoyed during the war were effectively placed on the back burner until later in the century. For the time being, "Father Knows Best" was on TV and Dr. Spock was telling mothers how to be mothers. Sadly, the Golden Age of Women's Sports was over.

THE DRIVE FOR EQUALITY—THE MODERN ERA

It wasn't until the 1960s and 1970s that women once again began to fight for their right to participate equally in sports opportunities, both as amateurs and professionals. They watched from the sidelines as the world of men's athletics mushroomed into the multibillion-dollar industry that it is today. This breakout into commercial and professional sports affected every level of competition, enabling thousands of men to compete in high-stakes college athletics and then go on to make their living as professional athletes.

When women first began banging at the door to this "sportsworld," they of course encountered plenty of opposition. At schools where they were able to get sanctioned support for teams, their budgets were characteristically anemic compared to the men's teams. Even at Vassar, a college that had helped create the very first sporting opportunities for women, the budget for men's athletics was twice that of women's in their very first coed year. Ironically, at this time the enrollment was still two-thirds women!

To a generation that had long ago forgotten women's achievements in the 1920s and 1930s, women once again had to prove that they were capable in athletics. Unfortunately, their opportunities to train and excell were limited. Women were still excluded from many sports in the Olympics, including pole vaulting, weight lifting, high hurdles, and all forms of team games except volleyball. In her 1965 book *Connotations of Movement in Sport and Dance*, Eleanor Metheny theorized that women were being excluded because society didn't want women competing in sports with the potential for body contact and the need to physically subdue an opponent. Once again, men were busy protecting women's reproductive organs and femininity!

Thankfully, the blossoming women's rights and civil rights movements were giving people the courage to ignore societal rules while they worked to change them. In 1967, Katherine Switzer entered the Boston Maraton as K. Switzer. Women were not allowed to run in the event, and when officials discovered "K" running the race, they tried to bodily remove her. She slipped past them, however, and ran right into the history books. Regardless of Katherine's successful finish, amateur athletic organizations still did not believe women were capable of running distance events. It was not until 1972 that women were "allowed" to compete in marathons.

The next great emancipating event for sporting women came on September 20, 1973. Billie Jean King had agreed to duel it out with one of the greatest self-proclaimed male chauvinists of all time, Bobby Riggs. What women wanted was the right to compete against each other in professional tennis; what they got was a battle of the sexes. Billie Jean won the three-out-of-five-set match in three straight. She went on to set world records of her own (including twenty Wimbledon championships), and then to break ground in advocacy for women's sports. It is largely because of her efforts that women are today earning lucrative purses in well-publicized tennis events.

The greatest leap forward came in 1972 when an educational amendment called Title IX was enacted. In a nutshell, Title IX prohibited discrimination on the basis of sex in educational institutions that receive federal funds (thus including most of the institutions in the country). No longer could a school deny women the right to facilities, budgets, coaches, uniforms, and so forth. It did not say that institutions had to match men and women's programs dollar for dollar, however, nor was it intended to benefit just women. Under Title IX, men could also lobby to form teams that often didn't exist, such as men's field hockey or volleyball.

Title IX was a monumental landmark, but as we have seen in recent years, it is neither perfect nor untouchable. Women's sports suffered a setback in 1987 when courts basically ruled that schools did not have to comply with Title IX. As a result, many institutions are dropping the reforms they had adopted, which tells us that although it may sometimes feel like we are in another Golden Age, we may be only at a peak in the undulating saga of women and sports in America. The value of history is to remind us to take none of our freedoms for granted.

WHO'S INFORMING US TODAY?

In the last ten to fifteen years, the fitness boom has transformed the way we live. Both women and men are heeding the advice of medical doctors, exercise physiologists, and psychologists who say that regular exercise can only help to improve the quality of our lives. More research has been done on exercise in the past decade than in all previous decades combined, and much of it is finding its way into the popular press. Audiences religiously read sports medicine columns in newspapers and in magazines devoted to various sports from waterskiing to ultramarathoning.

Because research has traditionally focused on male subjects, much of what is being written about women today is brand new information. Even as you read this book, our culture is in the process of shaping its opinion of active women. In large part, it will be based on the findings in these studies. Unfortunately, not all research reporting is accurate. Hungry for information, columnists sometimes run with stories prematurely, giving impressions that are not only misleading but actually dangerous. In many ways, we are not so different from our predecessors who read warnings in the popular press a century ago. We still tend to believe the printed word.

In 1982, a study was done on a limited sample of women runners who were experiencing amenorrhea (loss of periods). The researchers found that all the women had evidence of bone loss in their spine, a factor that would presumably put them at risk for osteoporosis, which is a condition of weakened bones that can lead to bone breakage. This single, rather anomalous study created a furor. Alarmist articles in the popular press warned women that running would cause them to lose their periods and develop brittle bones. A Melpomene study with a larger sample of women refuted these findings. We argued that although some high-mileage runners are amenorrheic, it is not an automatic consequence of running. There are many other factors such as stress and diet that influence menstrual patterns. We fear that the correction may have come too late, however. Negative myths have uncanny staying power, especially with people who are predisposed to the notion. For those who never tried exercising, the negative headlines may have been enough to justify their sedentary lifestyle.

A similar situation occurred with a study of pregnant women. The articles had frightening headlines like "Vigorous Exercise Can Slow Fetal Heart Rate." Although the reporters go on to explain that the temporary slowdown did not seem to harm the mothers or the fetuses in the study, many women may not have read that far. The message came across loud and clear: Exercise endangers the health of your unborn child. Follow-up studies have found this assumption to be simplistic and erroneous.

Another case of misinterpreted findings followed the release of "Safety Guidelines for Women Who Exercise" by the American College of Obstetricians and Gynecologists (ACOG) in the spring of 1985. The guidelines recommended fifteen to sixty minutes of aerobic activity, three to five days per week, at 60 percent to 90 percent of aerobic capacity. Quite correctly, the guidelines cautioned women to build up to vigorous activity gradually: "A given level of intensity, duration, and frequency may be safe for a well-conditioned woman but hazardous for one who is deconditioned."

These guidelines were talking about minimum fitness levels for women who were just starting an exercise program, and were not directed to elite athletes or even recreational athletes. And yet some reporters missed these subtleties. Headlines such as "Docs Tell Women: Go Easy on Exercise" and "Curbs Urged on Exercise for Women" implied that women who were exercising more than three times a week were doing too much. This conclusion, of course, was not ACOG's intention, but we felt that a clarification was necessary. We consulted some of our national advisory board members and issued a press release coauthored by the Women's Sports Foundation. It stated: "There is no reason for women to limit their exercise to this small quantity. Recreational athletes may choose to exercise for much greater amounts and competitive athletes will need to."

These examples and others point to the need for more careful, judicious treatment of research findings in the popular press. The jury on women and exercise is still deliberating, and mistaken notions may lead women to sell their exercise bikes and hang up their running shoes. Mothers reading this information are forming opinions that may affect how readily they accept their daughter's interest in athletics. One study found that 32 percent of college athletes show some form of eating disorder behavior (such as binge eating, vomiting, or laxative use). This study was widely reported in the press, and has led to the impression that women athletes have problems with food. Again, Melpomene has found that these responses may have been overstated. In a carefully controlled study of 229 athletes in 1989, we found only a 4.7 percent incidence of eating disorders, a far less daunting figure.

Beside the medical tug-of-war that pulls women into and out of exercise, there are social factors that can exert even stronger pulls. One of the longest-running campaigns to discredit women athletes revolves around the question of femininity. In a Women's Sports Foundation study conducted in 1985, 57 percent of the 1,682 women surveyed agreed that society still forces women to choose between femininity and athletics. Although it is now known that women athletes have high self-esteem and live happy lives, people still tend to question their motives for playing sports.

Women in sports that require physical strength or developed muscles are particularly suspect. Gender testing in Olympic athletes is a blatant example of the obsessive suspicion that plagues women. It seems that society is still more comfortable with women who participate in "acceptable" sports; that is, those that emphasize feminine characteristics such as grace and beauty. Olympic broadcasters, for instance, are more likely to make "sweethearts" out of gymnasts and figure skaters than women shot-putters or body builders. In a sad kind of "apologetic" behavior, many women in suspect sports go to great lengths to prove their femininity by wearing conspicuous jewelry or makeup on the playing field.

A few brave souls in the women's sports movement have begun to sweep aside the euphemisms that obscure this issue. They suggest that concerns about femininity are a smoke screen for a far more complex and pervasive fear—homophobia, or the irrational fear of homosexuality. Indeed, there are lesbians in women's sports, just as there are in every segment of society. But the closet seems to be larger and blacker here, even harder to open than in other arenas of modern life. Unfortunately, living in the closet robs the women's sports movement of much of its power. Consider, for instance, how damaging it is for a college coach to be accused of being a lesbian. Regardless of whether the gossip is true or false, she often has a harder time recruiting athletes, and she may even lose influence with those who hold the purse strings. This threat alone is enough to force women into "apologetic" behaviors and, not incidentally, to keep men in a position of undue power.

As long as lesbianism is synonymous with shame, women will continue to be blackmailed by inappropriate or unfounded rumors. Once again, we are called to disarm the myths so they cannot be used against us. Honest women like Martina Navratilova prove to everyone that sexual preference is not what's important about an athlete; sheer, miraculous talent is the focus. If we could learn to be proud of all women athletes, regardless of their sexual preference, we could also learn how to accept other groups of now "invisible" women in sports. Perhaps our new image of athletes could include large women, minority women, old women, and disabled women. Just think of how this viewpoint would expand our pool of talent!

Innuendos and distorted facts are powerful forces in our information society. Unfortunately, they have the power to discourage us from activities that could improve our health and change the very core of our beings. To avoid being manipulated, we all need to listen more critically, ask more questions, and find out where we can go for information that we can trust. Throughout this book, we encourage you to walk completely around an issue until you see it from all sides. The latest reports are only a step in the process of understanding women and physical activity. They may or may not prove to be true as time goes by. With this in mind, we hope you'll listen to the "experts" with a grain of salt. Next time you hear someone say "Stop exercising," consider the source, consider the times, and by all means, *ask for a second opinion!*

T W O

BODY IMAGE/BODY MIRAGE

Body image is the picture of our physical selves that we carry in our mind's eye. Often, this image has little resemblance to how we actually look. Our attitudes, perceptions, and value judgments overlay the mental picture, giving us an emotional rather than an objective view.

Consider Lisa, a forty-six-year-old mother who's feeling particularly fat and frumpy one morning. When her seventeen-year-old daughter says, "Mom, you look really pretty," Lisa sarcastically rolls her eyes. "Mom, I'm serious," her daughter says. "Why do you believe me when I tell you something doesn't look good, but always think I'm kidding when I honestly try to compliment you? I think you need some help with your body image."

How accurate is your body image? Is it possible to change the way you feel about your body? In this chapter, we'll introduce you to some of the latest research on body image and help you sort out what is truthful and what is unrealistic about your own body image. We'll also look at the prejudices and beliefs that many of us have about different body shapes, and see how these perceptions can wound your self-esteem. Finally, we'll investigate ways that you can erase the "negative tapes," and learn to love the body you have.

Before you read the chapter, you may want to check out some of your current beliefs by taking the following quiz. The questions reflect both opinions and facts. The test will not be scored, because there are no right or wrong answers to the opinion questions. Instead, your answers will serve to document what you currently believe about body image. After you finish the chapter, take the test again to see if your perception has changed.

	Agree	Neutral	Disagree
If you have ever been fat, it is very difficult to lose a "fat body" image.	❏	❏	❏
It is possible to be too thin.	❏	❏	❏
Body fat measurements are the best indicators of fitness and fatness.	❏	❏	❏
An ideal body fat percentage for a forty-year-old woman is 19 percent.	❏	❏	❏
Women's perceptions of their bodies are often inaccurate.	❏	❏	❏
The media is responsible for an increased number of eating disorders.	❏	❏	❏
Women are constantly encouraged to make changes in their appearance.	❏	❏	❏
Thin women are more likely to attract men and get better jobs.	❏	❏	❏
Athletes who are thin perform better than those who are heavier.	❏	❏	❏
Preschool children choose thin playmates over fatter ones.	❏	❏	❏
By the time girls are in high school, they are more likely than boys to be dissatisfied with their body shape.	❏	❏	❏
High school girls of average weight are more likely to go to college than girls who are obese.	❏	❏	❏
Men like women fatter than we think they do.	❏	❏	❏
I feel better about my body than I did five years ago.	❏	❏	❏
I could never be too thin.	❏	❏	❏
I have favorable memories of the way I looked as a child.	❏	❏	❏
I constantly worry about my weight or my eating patterns.	❏	❏	❏
Friends are more important to me than the way I look.	❏	❏	❏

	Agree	Neutral	Disagree
When people tell me "I'm looking good," I assume they mean I look thin.	❏	❏	❏
Losing five or ten pounds will not do much to improve my health.	❏	❏	❏
Exercising will increase my fitness level; it may also *increase* my weight.	❏	❏	❏
I can accurately estimate calories in most foods.	❏	❏	❏
There are "good" and "bad" foods.	❏	❏	❏
I sometimes say I am "bad" when I eat sweets or junk food.	❏	❏	❏

Body image—how you perceive your physical self—is a complex part of your self-image that begins to form in infancy and evolves throughout life. Your idea of your body is a composite of the attitudes of your parents, your classmates, and later, your adult peers. The attitudes of those around you, however, are usually reflections of how the society at large views different body shapes.

HOW SOCIETY SHAPES OUR BODY IMAGE

In some societies, a large, rounded woman is admired for her fertile body. A large man may be envied because of his ability to feed himself when food is scarce. Today, in our largely overfed culture, Americans are gripped by a feverish obsession to be thin and fit. Thinness is associated with high social class, with success, and with the ability to attract a man. The standard of female beauty has become more narrowly defined and restrictive, making it nearly impossible to be thin enough, fit enough, or young enough. Society, in effect, keeps moving the finish line farther and farther back, ensuring that most of us will never attain the unrealistic "ideal."

Psychologist Bean Robinson, Ph.D., writing in the February 1985 *Melpomene Report*, reminds us that "thinness has not always been viewed with such universal fervor and longing. In earlier times, from approximately 1400–1900, the more voluptuous abundant female figure was seen as the ideal type." Western taste keeps changing, giving us at least three different ideal body types for women since about 1500. The first was tummy-centered and often quite fat. William Bennet and Joel Gurin, authors of the book, *The Dieters Dilemma, Eating Less and Weighing More*, call her the "reproductive figure."

Between 1650 and 1700, taste changed throughout Europe to a new ideal, which was rather plump and all bosom and bottom; her narrow, often-corseted waist was designed to emphasize these ample endowments. Bennet and Gurin label this type the "maternal figure." Then, rather rapidly between 1910 and 1920, this full-blown female figure lost favor within Anglo-American culture and was replaced by a tubular, lean, and slender figure with minimal breast and buttocks and little remnant of the promising, reproductive tummy. Bennet and Gurin call her the "sexual free agent."

While there has been some fluctuation of ideal body weight and shape in the twentieth century, the general trend has been toward even thinner models. A 1930s magazine titled *Fitness*, which included several articles devoted to women and physical fitness, portrays healthy women who are clearly twenty pounds heavier than those we would find in a 1989 publication. Today, those magazines devoted to skiing, running, tennis, or cycling all use models for their covers who look as if they are on an 800-calorie-a-day diet. Even the *Playboy* centerfold has lost twenty-five pounds in the last twenty years. She is now 18 percent less than what would be considered a medical ideal or normal for her age and height. In a short span of time, we have moved from at least a gently rounded figure to the woman whom nutritionist Julie Jones, Ph.D., described as "the backless, frontless, buttless wonder."

OUR NATIONAL OBSESSION WITH THINNESS

As women, we are constantly encouraged to work toward this lean, tubular shape, even though it may be structurally impossible or even medically dangerous for us to be so skinny. Losing weight has become synonymous with "taking care of yourself," or "not letting yourself go." Next time you are on the checkout line at the supermarket, scan the headline articles of leading women's magazines. Notice how many magazines have a "makeover" that stresses weight loss. Almost all of these magazines feature dieting articles every month except December, when they emphasize the psychological importance of food! Further, our obsession seems to be growing. Between 1958 and 1968, 17.1 percent of the articles in six popular women's magazines were about dieting and losing weight; this figure increased to 29.6 percent between 1969 and 1978.

At Melpomene, we're concerned about the impact of this trend on young women. In 1986, Laurel Millin of the University of California asked almost five hundred schoolgirls in San Francisco about their dieting patterns. Almost half the nine-year-olds and 80 percent of the ten- and eleven-year-olds said they were dieting to lose weight. Of seventeen-year-old students, 89 percent said they were on diets. Millin reported that while 58 percent of the girls surveyed said they were overweight, only 17 percent actually were. The number of the girls who reported binge eating increased steadily with age and all the eighteen-year-olds said they currently used vomiting, laxatives, fasting, or diet pills to help them control their weight.

To understand what motivates this destructive behavior, think about what it means to be thin in America. "You can never be too rich or too thin," the saying goes. And indeed, thinness seems to be equated with material success and happiness. Look back at your responses to the questions regarding thinness and fatness. Did you say that thin women were more likely to attract men and get better jobs? There are research reports that confirm your suspicion. An attractive (thin) woman *is* more likely to attract a man and have access to better job opportunities. Is it any wonder that girls and women have become so preoccupied with weight?

THE CONSEQUENCES OF BEING OVERWEIGHT

In a society where thinness is rewarded, being large can be both a social and an economic liability. A large person is often seen as being out of control and socially undesirable. Large people are frequently described as lazy, awkward, weak-willed, and dumb.

Lenore Manells and Jean Mayer, nutritionists at the Harvard School of Public Health, reported that obese girls attending a weight reduction camp in Massachusetts showed personality characteristics that were strikingly similar to those of ethnic and racial minorities. It seems that the oppression of prejudice, regardless of its nature, leaves emotional scars that are hard to erase.

Though it's frightening to consider, statistics show that negative stereotyping may be locking large women out of colleges. In another study conducted with Helen Canning of the Harvard School of Public Health, Mayer reported that, "In a large suburban community, 51.9 percent of the nonobese high school women went to college the year after graduation as compared with only 31.6 percent of the obese. The obese and nonobese women did *not* differ on objective measures of intellectual ability and achievement or on the percentage who applied for college admission." Canning and Mayer concluded that college admission discrimination could contribute to the obese not realizing their educational or economic potential.

Knowing that body shape can have such an enormous impact, is it really shocking or surprising that some young mothers start their children on diets when they are only six months old? We at Melpomene can't help but wonder what connection these kiddie diets might have to the rising prevalence of eating disorders over the last ten years.

WHEN DO WE DEVELOP BODY IMAGE?

Stop and reflect on your own body image. When were you first aware of how you looked? Chances are you were aware of your body image even before you knew how you felt about yourself as a person. You may have noticed that your body had an impact on the way people looked at you and treated you.

What other people say makes a difference at a very early age. Perhaps you remember getting messages as a little girl such as, "Aren't you clever!" "You run fast for someone so young!" "You look pretty now that you're all dressed up!" Fewer women have favorable memories of hearing, "My, how strong you are!" "You're going to be big and tall!" Such observations were usually reserved for little boys. Somehow, even at a young age, we knew that it was not flattering to be called "strong" or to have too much athletic prowess.

How did these early messages affect how we would feel about our bodies twenty years later? There are not many studies that look *prospectively* (projecting into the future) at the complex issues of how body image is formed. At Melpomene, we are involved in a unique study that looks at the socialization patterns of children at early ages. We are fortunate to be able to work with mothers who have already participated in two of our earlier studies on exercise and pregnancy. We already know something about the lifestyles of these women, and about their attitudes toward physical activity. Half of the women we interviewed hadn't exercised at all during pregnancy; the others had run or swum regularly both before and during pregnancy. We were initially interested in finding out what impact, if any, a mother's exercise history might have on how she socializes her child.

Early results indicate that mothers who were more physically active were more likely to describe their children in terms of skills and personality rather than by body shape and size. Unfortunately, this highlight runs counter to the norm. Most people heavily emphasize body shape and size when describing kids, and, as a result, youngsters become aware of being fat or thin at a very early age. Studies show that by preschool, children are already choosing thin children as playmates over fatter ones, with obvious implications for self-esteem. The fat child needs other very positive input to believe that she is "okay"; it is usually not until a person has reached adulthood, if at all, that she can ignore the societal pressure to be thin.

In a Montreal study conducted by psychologists Beverly Katz Mendelson and Donna Romano White, thirty-six subjects ages seven and a half to twelve years old completed a self-esteem and body-esteem questionnaire. Sixteen of the subjects—eleven girls and five boys—were more than 15 percent overweight. These children had a lower opinion of their bodies and personal appearance than normal-weight children, suggesting that they had already accepted the cultural norm that says thinner is better. The authors also found that, "Children who are dissatisfied with personal appearances are also dissatisfied with aspects of their lives unrelated to looks, aspects such as intellectual and school status, behavior, and anxiety." The overweight children did not yet suffer from lower self-esteem, however. They were still able to say "I don't like my body very well, but I like myself." In subsequent studies with more subjects, Mendelson and White found that this good self-esteem doesn't last very long. By later adolescence, overweight girls were much more likely than normal-weight girls to develop low self-esteem related to body size.

Another very interesting study of 406 children enrolled in grades four to six in a midwestern community was conducted by Susan Ferencz Stager and Peter Burke. In this study, both girls and boys used the same adjectives to describe fat children, including, "less good looking," "more often teased," and "having fewer friends." Some children saw themselves in the fat child stereotype, even if they themselves were not overweight. The children who identified most strongly with the fat child stereotype had the lowest self-esteem. Stager and Burke also found that the skinny child stereotype was viewed favorably. In fact, when compared to a study done ten years earlier, the skinny child stereotype had become even more favorable.

Because the negative consequences of being overweight seem to get worse as a child gets older, Mendelson and White suggest enrolling children in a program to reduce weight before their overall self-concept is damaged. Today, children as young as eight years old can enter programs designed to reduce weight and revamp unhealthy lifestyles. Some of the programs are well-conceived and take into consideration the psychological as well as the nutritional aspects of being overweight.

Before enrolling your child in such a program, however, you'll want to determine whether the child is actually overweight, and by what degree. It may be that you, as a parent, are more concerned than your child, and perhaps more concerned than you need to be. Before you call attention to the problem, consider the impact that it will have on your child's self-concept, and be sure that the problem is worth the risk.

PRESSURES INCREASE IN HIGH SCHOOL

If the growing number of weight-conscious children in grade school disturbs you, wait until you see the statistics on high school kids! By high school, the obsession with weight and dieting becomes extremely common, especially among girls. In 1983, Nancy Storz, a faculty member of the School of Nursing at the University of Pennsylvania, and Walter Greene, member of the Health Education faculty at Temple University, looked at body weight, body image, and perception of fad diets in adolescent girls. They studied fourteen- to eighteen-year-olds living in middle-class rural and suburban areas near Philadelphia. Of the 203 participants, 83 percent said they wanted to lose weight, 14 percent wanted to gain, and only 2 percent wanted to maintain their current weight. "Of the 169 subjects desiring weight loss, 94 (56 percent) wanted to lose at least 10 percent of their actual body weight in spite of the fact that 62 percent actually fell within the average range for body weight."

Boys don't seem to be nearly as dissatisfied with their body shape as girls are. In a Gallup Poll in which 59 percent of teenage girls said they wanted to lose weight, 52 percent of the boys said that their weight was fine, and 28 percent wanted to gain weight. For girls, this perceived need to lose weight might be related to the natural changes of puberty. Many girls feel that the onset of menstruation and the swelling of their breasts is something that simply happens to them; though they may worry about the timing of these events, there's not much they can do to control them. To a great extent, additional weight is also part of maturing, but girls seem to view it differently. Along with the rest of society, they see body weight as something that a disciplined person should be able to manipulate and control. Perhaps weight control steals center stage because this is the one area where adolescent girls feel they can influence their body.

The shape many girls are striving for is not necessarily a healthy one. The Gallup Poll mentioned above showed that girls who were asked to choose their ideal weight inevitably chose one that was 10 percent below the recommended "ideal" weight. All the girls, whether they were within recommended ranges or not, described themselves as being 10 percent overweight. This tendency to define oneself as fatter than is objectively true persists throughout most of a woman's life.

A woman's perception of her own body is often based on what she thinks someone else finds attractive. A need to conform and therefore be accepted may be most important during high school and college years. In a survey of five hundred college-age men and women, Paul Rozin and April Fallon of the University of Pennsylvania found that women say they are heavier than what they think men find attractive. Moreover, they would prefer to weigh even less than the ideal body weight they think men would choose. Are these women seeking the media stereotype of anorexic thinness? Interestingly, when men were questioned, they said that they actually liked somewhat heavier women. In other studies where men and women were asked to identify attractive body sizes, the men viewed a greater range of weights as potentially attractive. They were also more tolerant of their own excess weight than the women were.

HOW ACCURATE IS YOUR BODY IMAGE?

Clearly, many of our attitudes about our bodies are formed when we are younger and are shaped by what we think is appropriate or expected of us. There seems to be a separate set of expectations for men and women, and therefore, our gender may determine whether we are tolerant or appreciative of our bodies. To examine your current feelings, try the following exercise: Look at the drawings below and choose the one you think best reflects your body size. Now select the body size you would like to have. Are they the same?

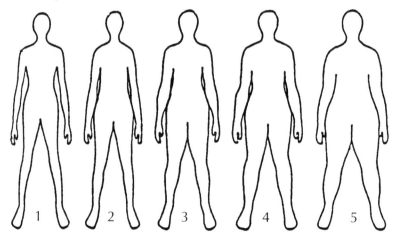

These drawings represent bodies that are (1) 20 percent underweight, (2) 10 percent underweight, (3) average weight, (4) 10 percent overweight, and (5) 20 percent overweight. If you chose one of the underweight figures for your "ideal," you are not alone. In one of our recent studies, we asked physically active women whose average age was thirty-two to do just what you did. Thirty-eight percent of the respondents said they would like to be 20 percent underweight and an additional 44 percent said they would like to be 10 percent underweight. Only 14 percent thought that an average-size body was desirable!

In a similar study of college-age women, researchers Miller, Coffman, and Linke found that 63 percent of the women overestimated their own size. The desired weight for women in the study was 116 pounds or 14 pounds less than their reported weight. Look again at the silhouettes. Did you say you wanted a body that was 10 percent underweight? How accurate do you think you are in assessing your true body shape? To test your self-perception, ask both a male and female friend to select the body shape most like yours.

Here's another question. Do you consider yourself underweight, slightly underweight, just right, slightly overweight, or overweight? Thirty-five percent of the Melpomene respondents considered themselves "just right" with regard to weight. Sixty percent felt they were overweight to some degree. When we looked at their actual weight and height, we found that most fell within the normal weight range.

If you chose a small body size, which may be extremely difficult or even impossible for you to achieve, it might be time to start looking at this issue more realistically. If you are among those who would give anything to lose ten pounds, consider the possibility that the effort required to lose it may not bring the desired results. Many experts agree that losing or gaining five or ten pounds does not make much of a difference in appearance.

WHICH PARTS DO YOU LIKE BEST?

If you are dissatisfied with your body, perhaps it is not completely a weight issue. The way you feel about your body as a whole stems from the way you feel about various parts of your body. Rating your arms, legs, face, and so forth in the following questionnaire may help you discover why you are pleased or frustrated with your body as a whole.

Consider each item listed below and circle the number that best represents your feelings according to the following scale:

	Have strong negative feelings and wish change could somehow be made	Don't like but can put up with	Have no particular feelings one way or the other	Am satisfied	Consider myself fortunate
1. Hair	1	2	3	4	5
2. Teeth	1	2	3	4	5
3. Eyes	1	2	3	4	5
4. Ears	1	2	3	4	5
5. Nose	1	2	3	4	5
6. Skin	1	2	3	4	5
7. Overall facial attractiveness	1	2	3	4	5
8. Arms	1	2	3	4	5
9. Breasts/chest	1	2	3	4	5
10. Shoulders	1	2	3	4	5
11. Abdomen	1	2	3	4	5
12. Hips	1	2	3	4	5
13. Waist	1	2	3	4	5
14. Upper legs (thighs)	1	2	3	4	5
15. Lower legs (calves)	1	2	3	4	5
16. Body build	1	2	3	4	5
17. Posture	1	2	3	4	5
18. Weight	1	2	3	4	5
19. Height	1	2	3	4	5
20. Level of physical fitness	1	2	3	4	5
21. Energy level	1	2	3	4	5

22. Overall, how satisfied are you with the way you look?

Just as men and women differ on their perceptions of weight, they also have very different criteria for overall body satisfaction. Psychologist Beavens found that adolescent girls want to change specific parts of their bodies whereas boys are concerned with overall body appearance. You can check for yourself by asking your teenage daughter or friend to complete the body parts scale above.

Your peer group and social environment may also have something to do with your level of satisfaction. In Melpomene studies, we found that girls attending suburban and private high schools tended to be less satisfied with their bodies than those attending large public high schools in cities. While the data need to be explored in more depth, conversations with respondents suggest that the larger, more economically diverse schools had broader definitions of acceptable body shapes.

Unfortunately, we don't seem to get any better at accurately judging our body size as we get older; women of all ages misrepresented their true size in our studies. On the other hand, men seem to have an almost unrealistic satisfaction with their bodies as reported by Rozin and Fallon in their study of five hundred college students. This kind of positive body image, while it may distort reality, also has obvious psychological benefits.

Men and women differed significantly in their responses to the body parts questionnaire that you completed. For a 1986 Melpomene study on body image, we asked a sample of physically active men and women from a running race to complete the questionnaire, as well as a nonactive comparison group. In both groups, we were able to predict the sex of a respondent just by looking at the number of positive responses to the assessment of body parts. Men frequently chose the most positive response, "I consider myself fortunate," while women were rarely more positive than "I am satisfied." How do your responses compare? You may also wish to use this questionnaire with a male friend to verify our results for yourself.

Within the group of runners, women were more likely to say that body parts not associated with shape were the body parts they like best (i.e., eyes, hair, and overall facial attractiveness). The body parts liked least were thighs (53 percent of the respondents), abdomen (34 percent), and hips (33 percent). Since these women are physically active, perhaps it is not surprising that calves were ranked as a body part liked best by 45 percent of the respondents.

THE STRUGGLE TO "IMPROVE"

MAKEUP

Do most women really spend time worrying about how certain pieces of their body look? If we don't, says our society, perhaps we should. Think about a typical hour of network TV. You may see twelve commercials that urge you to fix what's "wrong" with you by using products such as hair coloring, facial cosmetics, hair removers, dry skin lotion, tummy tighteners, artificial nails, colored contact lenses, and breath fresheners. Advertisers imply that if we simply work on one piece of ourselves at a time, we will realize all our dreams for love and success.

The campaign waged by the cosmetics industry reaches girls at an early age. From their teenage years on, women are encouraged to spend large sums of money on their faces. The illusion is that skillfully applied makeup can hide or eliminate your imperfections so that you are more attractive and desirable. Consider Sandra. She spends a minimum of forty-five minutes each morning decorating her face. When she is finished she is pleased with the results and feels much more confident to begin her day as a lawyer. "It makes a big difference professionally if I look well," she says. Jackie, on the other hand, spends a brief five minutes giving her face only minimal attention. She says that her competency is more important than her looks. Both may be right. Jackie's self-confidence in her natural looks, however, saves her more than an hour each day. She says she prefers to spend that time reading or exercising.

COSMETIC SURGERY

Most women, as they age, learn to accept the physical features that are not related to weight. Some, however, continue to focus their dissatisfaction on a long nose, sagging eyes, or small breasts. More and more of these women are considering cosmetic surgery as a way to "improve" the parts they like least. Their desire seems linked to a notion we are all led to believe: that beauty is only a matter of effort, and that perfection is possible if only we can find the means to achieve it.

Have you ever personally wondered about changing a body part through surgery? The variety of woman seriously considering it may surprise you. At Melpomene, we've noticed that within the last five years, women are talking more openly about this option. For the first time, for instance, we've been asked to include cosmetic surgery as a topic in our yearly body image conference.

In some cases, cosmetic surgery can make a positive difference. Someone who has been truly unhappy with her nose may find that she is happier and more confident as well as more attractive following surgery. Jane, for example, had been uncomfortable with her nose for as long as she could remember. Some newspaper ads plus an article in a magazine convinced her to explore the possibility of surgery in more detail. While she was somewhat embarrassed to be thinking about something that seemed so vain, she still wanted to know the facts so she could make a wise choice. Not only did she interview several physicians and check out the details of cost and probable outcome but she also talked with several women who had undergone the same procedure. After a year of asking questions and weighing outcomes, Jane finally scheduled her operation. She reports that the change was just what she had hoped, and that her self-confidence has blossomed as a result.

Sarah's story is quite different. Her husband and friends scoffed when she talked about wanting a face-lift. "You look young and wonderful as you are," they told her. But Sarah was determined and had high expectations for her surgery. "The surgical team was honest in telling me that in my case the improvements would be minimal," Sarah admitted later, "but I still wanted to try it." Unfortunately, Sarah had surgical complications. A new, crooked smile was only one of the negative results that made Sarah angry that she had decided to try to look younger.

Why do women consider cosmetic surgery? Some people believe that the desire to change your appearance must be rooted in deep psychological problems. Psychologists Judith Burk, Seymour Zelen, and Edward Terino, associated with the California School of Professional Psychology, believe it may be more straightforward than that. According to their tests, they describe the typical surgery candidate as a woman who is "average in terms of general self-esteem, but whose physical self-esteem is lower than average and who seeks the practical solution of cosmetic surgery because of inconsistencies in her self-concept."

Basically, they suggest that a woman has surgery because she has one body part that she likes less than others. Cosmetic surgery is just one of three possible ways she might deal with her dissatisfaction: She can begin to see the body part as less important, she can continue to let it bother her but not do anything, or she can schedule surgery. In their experience, they have seen "stable improvement in esteem of the body as well as the operated body part over time following surgery."

Cosmetic surgery has also been the answer for many women who want some form of breast reconstruction after surgery for breast cancer. It took Maggie four years to decide to have breast reconstruction. Her physicians recommended she wait two years following her mastectomy to be sure there were no additional lumps. During that time she became increasingly uncomfortable with her prosthesis. "I was often in a swimsuit, and prostheses were really a bother."

When first exploring the possibility of surgery, she asked for recommendations from two of her friends in a mastectomy support group. She then arranged a session in which she and her husband were able to ask questions of one of the physicians and his team. Maggie felt the team presented excellent information, but she also called back the next day to get some additional questions answered. Because she felt very comfortable with her decision, the time lapse between this visit and the surgery was only six weeks.

The first surgery in the two-step process took two hours, and Maggie was in the hospital less than two days. Her pain was minimal and she felt well on her way to complete recovery in one week. She completed her final surgery as an outpatient four months later. Maggie reported that her major complaint was being tired, but that recovery seemed very easy.

She is extremely pleased with the results. "It feels like I have a breast again!" She thinks that the time between her mastectomy and the decision to have surgery was critical for her. She doesn't think all women should have this surgery, but she has become an advocate due to her positive experience.

While some of us may never consider cosmetic surgery, most of us will continue to try to "improve" our physical appearance in other ways. Sometimes we don't consciously realize what it is about ourselves that we consider most important. Take a few seconds to try a simple but revealing exercise. The directions are easy: *describe yourself.*

If you are like the majority of women, you answered with physical attributes rather than character descriptions. You mentioned features that you feel are distinctive, or even central, to who you are. Ironically, regardless of other personal descriptors, you probably also mentioned weight.

LOSING WEIGHT

The serious impact that weight has on many women's lives became startlingly clear in a 1984 survey by *Glamour* magazine. Women were asked which they would prefer: (1) a date with a man they admire, (2) seeing an old friend, (3) a promotion or success at work, or (4) losing weight. The greatest percentage chose losing weight. In a 1987 *Ms.* magazine survey, losing weight was not a number-one priority but 64.4 percent agreed with the statement, "I would like myself better if I were thinner." Obviously, weight and body shape, or rather, a woman's *perception* of her shape, is a critical factor in how she feels about herself as a person.

Many woman see themselves as overweight and undesirable when they are actually within the ideal weight range for their age. But who decides what is ideal weight? Quantitative data on weight, both actual and ideal, first appeared around the turn of the century. The first ideal weight tables, compiled in 1912, were the work of the Association of Life Insurance Medical Directors of America and were derived from a survey of life insurance policyholders. They set standards of height and weight by bone structure using the groups with the lowest death rates as the ideal. These tables, which were updated and revised in 1931, 1943, 1959, and 1982, have become the standards most doctors and the general public usually choose to determine relative fatness or thinness. Although these standards are open to question, millions of Americans are still relying on them to see how they measure up! Until the latest revision, the actual weight of the American population was increasing, and the ideal weight proposed by medical actuaries was decreasing.

There were also interesting differences between men and women. By 1974, men's actual weight was greater than the recommended standards, but women's actual weight was less. The major difference is that many women continually control their weight through restricted eating whereas men are less likely to do so.

Dr. Reubin Andres, clinical director of the Gerontology Research Center of the National Institute on Aging, contends that the Metropolitan Life Charts are "too high for young people, too low for middle-aged and older, and just right for those in their early forties." Gerontology experts tell us that it is reasonable for our weight to increase as we age. Most of us will not fit into our wedding dress twenty-five years later. One Melpomene Institute volunteer said that she had only recently given away clothes she had worn when she was forty-seven and several pounds lighter. Now fifty-three, and still very trim and athletic, Miriam has finally become comfortable with her new weight and decided that the clothes will never fit again. Unfortunately, many women are not as accepting of their normal shifts in body weight that come with aging.

DIETING: THE NATIONAL PASTIME

Living up to the standards of ideal weight can be a lifelong struggle for many women. Although figures vary according to the study or survey quoted, somewhere between 40 percent and 50 percent of American women are on a diet of some sort at any given time. Yet many women who are on a diet are concerned with a five- or ten-pound loss rather than losses of twenty pounds or more. The loss of five or ten pounds will have few, if any, health benefits.

Wayne Calloway, M.D., an obesity specialist at the Mayo Clinic, has spoken about the healthy obese. He suggests that chronic unhappiness associated with repeated attempts at weight control may shorten your life. And there is little reason to believe that preoccupation with weight diminishes with age. In a longitudinal study of people over age sixty-two, researchers Ruth Streigel-Moore, Lisa Silberstein, and Judith Rodin report that "the second greatest personal concern expressed by women in the sample, following memory loss, was change in body weight."

It is frequently this preoccupation, rather than a therapeutic need to lose weight, that encourages dieting behavior. Melpomene studies indicate that women who diet are far less satisfied with their bodies than those who do not.

How often do you diet? If you are among the smaller percentage of

American women who can say "never," you will want to read this section to gain a better understanding of friends who are always dieting. On the other hand, if you sometimes or frequently diet, this section may help you evaluate whether or not you really need to diet and what you should expect.

When you decide you need to diet are you talking about a formal plan or something as simple as restricting snacks? Look at the following choices and identify the methods you would choose to reduce weight.

POPULAR WAYS OF REDUCING WEIGHT (NOT ALL RECOMMENDED)

Decrease size of portions
Eliminate carbohydrates
Avoid sweets
Count calories
Reduce fat intake
Eliminate snacks
Increase physical activity
Try a popular diet
Purge
Enroll in a weight reduction program
Fast
Increase caffeine intake
Start to smoke, or increase number of cigarettes smoked

THE TRUTH ABOUT OBESITY

Is there a good weight reduction diet? Some of the choices listed above are obviously more healthy than others, yet all are methods currently used by American women. What is the long-term success rate of dieting? Kelly Brownell, a professor in the department of psychiatry at the University of Pennsylvania, who has gained prominence in both research and writing about issues related to weight, says "if one defines successful treatment as return to ideal body weight and maintenance for five years, a person is more likely to recover from almost any form of cancer than from obesity."

Brownell's excellent paper, "Understanding and Treating Obesity," suggests that we need to look carefully at the studies linking obesity with health problems. Media "experts" and many physicians would have us believe that even ten extra pounds will make us more susceptible to long-term health problems. Granted, there may be health risks related to obesity, but it is not clear that obesity per se should always be blamed for medical problems that a large person may encounter. Interestingly, Brownell feels that the worst dangers of obesity may not be physical in nature. According to Brownell, "the psychological and social hazards of obesity may be as serious as the medical hazards."

Large people are often blamed for creating their own condition through gluttony or a simple lack of self-control. The fact is that many large people are very conscious of controlling their intake of calories. J. S. Garrow, a researcher who reviewed the most important studies on food intakes and body weight, found that in twelve out of thirteen studies, the obese subjects consumed the same amount of food or less than normal-weight subjects. Yet evidence reveals that even at similar intakes, large people face greater odds than normal-weight people when they try to lose weight.

Another popular myth is that large people could be thin if only they were physically active. This argument loses steam when you think about the thin people you know who aren't active at all. Why is it that they are able to eat all they want, live a sedentary lifestyle, and yet not become fat? The mounting body of evidence seems to indicate that the difference between fat people and thin people is not in their eating or activity patterns but rather in their biological makeup.

Your metabolism—the way your body burns fuel—is as individual as you are. In a carefully controlled study of normal-weight individuals, researchers Warwick, Toft, and Garrow found differences of 400 to 500 calories per day in resting metabolisms, which means that if two people watch TV, one may burn more calories per hour than the other simply by virtue of a faster metabolism. The greatest documented difference was 770 calories per day.

Researchers have also found that the amount of energy (or food) that a body needs in order to function at a given weight varies from person to person. After thoroughly reviewing the literature related to caloric intake

and weight, Sue Dyrenforth, Orland Wooley, and Susan Wooley concluded that "some women gain on 5,000 calories per day, some gain on
800."

Why do these differences occur? It is only recently that we have begun
to examine the role of heredity in relation to weight. Albert Stunkard and
colleagues at the University of Pennsylvania found that adopted children
had body weights that were more closely matched with their biological
parents than with their adopted parents. Maybe the old adage that says
we should look at our mothers to see how we will age has more truth to
it than we would like to admit! If your mother is someone who gains
weight even on a diet of only 800 or 1,000 calories, you too may have a
tendency to put on weight. If you then want to remove the weight, you'll
have some difficult decisions to make.

THE BEST DIETS: WADING THROUGH THE HYPE

Let's say you decide to diet at some time in your life. Your first task will
be to find the sensible diet (if there is one) amid the latest rash of weight-
loss scams that crowd supermarket checkouts and bookstore shelves. In
the Spring 1987 issue of the *Melpomene Journal*, nutritionist and author
Joan Vogel reviewed nine of the diet plans that you are likely to hear
about. She also gave some general guidelines that can help you avoid
bogus or even dangerous diets. Vogel warns against diets that usually
include one or all of the following tricks for quick weight loss:

- Eating fewer carbohydrates while consuming large amounts of fats
  and protein
- Eating only special foods and/or food supplements
- Drastically reducing the number of calories you consume

One of the main reasons these strategies tend to fail is because they
concentrate on what you shouldn't eat instead of recommending eating
habits that are healthy. Denying yourself certain foods is a quick fix rather
than a new lifestyle. Until you develop eating habits that you can comfortably live with for a lifetime, claims Vogel, any weight loss will be a

temporary one. Besides being just plain ineffective, some of these diets can also wreak havoc on your body.

When you are on a low-carbohydrate diet, your body will be burning fats for fuel. Since fats are not efficient producers of energy, waste products in the form of ketones are produced. This influx of ketones causes your kidneys to excrete more water and body fluids, while the rest of your body experiences a feeling of fatigue. Because you are eating fewer carbohydrates, chances are you are filling up with higher percentages of fats and proteins. The connection between these foods and higher blood cholesterol has been well-documented and publicized. What you may not have heard about is that high-fat, low-protein diets can also leave your body hungry for calcium and minerals such as iron.

Vogel warns, "The most destructive aspect of decreased protein is the breakdown of the body's muscle tissue to satisfy energy requirements. During this process, some of the body fat is lost but lean tissue or lean body mass is also reduced, causing a loss of strength."

The most extreme starvation diets are self-limiting. Usually the person quits because the side effects of fatigue, irritability, mood swings, and depression become unmanageable. One of the most devastating consequences of low-calorie diets is that they eventually reduce your resting metabolic rate, making it more difficult for you to burn off excess calories and lose weight.

Given this quick summary of the more blatant "quick-fix" diets (those that promise you'll lose five to ten pounds per week), are there any diets that can be recommended? According to Vogel, the two programs that are acceptable to most nutritionists are the Weight Watchers plan and the setpoint diet. These diets are selected because they encourage you to meet your requirements for calories and nutrients, while taking into account your sex, age, and amount of physical activity. Being able to choose your own food and work with food exchanges helps make these diets flexible and practical.

Even the best diet will reach a point of diminishing return when your body finally adapts to the smaller portions and lower number of calories. Basically, your body, which has evolved to survive all kinds of shortages, is tricked into believing that you are facing a famine. To keep you from losing too much weight, your body begins to burn fuel more slowly, stretching every serving you give it. Thanks to your new metabolic rate (15 percent to 30 percent lower than normal), you don't need to spend as many calories to accomplish a given amount of work. Naturally, and by design, this added efficiency makes it harder for you to lose pounds.

The same law of diminishing returns applies to physical exercise and weight loss. By the second year or third year of regular exercise, most women find that their body becomes accustomed to the extra energy drain. The body again becomes more efficient and doesn't need as many postrace milkshakes to replace the lost energy!

DO WE DIET BECAUSE WE'RE AFRAID?

Understanding how we gain and lose weight should help us to make informed choices about our eating habits. Unfortunately, however, even women who know the facts are likely to react irrationally when faced with their own weight gain. G. Terrance Wilson, a professor of psychology at Rutgers University, says that "no matter how 'perfect' a woman's figure may be, if she is told she looks fat, she will have an emotional reaction out of proportion to reality. On the other hand, if you tell her she looks thin or has lost weight, she will be inordinately pleased." Think about it. How often have you told someone that she looks fat?

Several women were discussing this issue at a Melpomene conference. One woman remarked:

> Only once did anyone tell me I looked fat. I was devastated, even though I knew it was not objectively true. I had gained about ten pounds and dreaded having someone say I looked heavier. Most of my friends are sensitive to the fact that I struggle with a distorted fat body image and have a tendency to think that thin is better. They would probably never tell me I looked heavier because they would know I would have the reaction Wilson describes.

The ironic part is that this woman had been a very thin runner and actually looked better at her new weight. Perhaps her deep-seated fear of being fat kept her from seeing the true image of herself in the mirror. Like most of us, she was programmed to believe that any weight gain, even if it is needed, is a dangerous trend.

Food and the struggle to control eating play a major role in the lives of many women. Consider Susan and Sally who struck up a conversation at their children's tennis meet. "Well, I finally did it," exclaimed Sally, "I signed up for Weight Watchers!" Susan, who didn't know Sally well, was somewhat surprised. Sally was a thin, attractive woman who did not look like she needed to lose weight. As they talked further, Sally revealed that she weighed herself two or three times every day, and spent at least an hour a day worrying about food. A pound or two was cause for concern; three or four pounds meant that she canceled plans to meet a friend for lunch. Although she always made up other excuses, the real reason for her change in plans was because she felt too fat.

Are women who are preoccupied with weight psychologically healthy? Mary Connors and Craig Johnson conclude that women who diet usually function well psychologically. Their studies indicate that weight-conscious women are a very diverse group, perhaps because this group encompasses such a large share of the American public.

As hard as it may be to accept, the fact is that we don't have a great deal of choice about the shape of our bodies. Ellen Goodman, syndicated columnist, has a novel approach to the problem. She suggests that we all grow several inches in the next year! We've considered offering a height-raising clinic at Melpomene; certainly if one can manipulate weight, height should also be susceptible to change! We immediately see the ridiculousness of this idea, yet for many women it's just as impossible to hope that they will one day wear a size seven or nine.

What if you are fat? What if you have tried fifteen sensible diets and they don't work? For many women, being large is a fact of life. An estimated 16 million women in America wear size sixteen or larger and therefore are labeled large or fat by society. One of these women, Alice Ansfield, who has an M.A. in clinical psychology, was tired of fighting prejudice and isolation; she was tired of focusing energy on the desire to be thin. She decided in 1984 that it was time to produce a positive, life-giving publication for large women like herself. *Radiance: The Magazine for Large Women* began as a four-page newsletter distributed to women attending an exercise class designed by and for larger women in Oakland, California. Two weeks later, it became a twenty-page publication with twenty-eight advertisers; by 1989 *Radiance* had grown to a sixty-page glossy magazine with a national readership of 140,000. *Radiance* features articles and stories "from women of all walks of life who have become experts on their own experiences as large woman living in an antifat world." The focus is on good health and positive self-esteem, a much-needed but hard-to-achieve commodity for many large women.

In an article written for the Winter 1988 *Melpomene Journal*, Ansfield (*Radiance* editor) and Pat Lyons report that discrimination and human isolation extract a heavy toll on the lives of most large women:

> Rather than be encouraged to inhabit the world as strong, healthy, vital people, many women of all sizes live instead in perpetual terror of gaining weight and measure their entire self-worth by the numbers on the scale. They postpone education, social life, creativity, career, and involvement in community activities, putting their energies instead into efforts to achieve an elusive, magical point in the future defined as "when I am thin." That many never reach that stage is a tragic story of wasted lives.

Of course, many women who are not technically obese are also held hostage by their preoccupation with weight; studies reveal that 60 percent to 80 percent of adult American women have this concern. Some recent commentaries suggest that the problem may be worsening among younger women. Dr. Francy Howland, New Haven psychiatrist and assistant professor at Yale Medical School, says, "I have yet to have one Yale woman tell me she does not have a problem with food."

How does a preoccupation with weight or a problem with food cross the line and become an eating disorder? Experts are unsure, but agree that an eating disorder is more than just dieting that has gotten out of control. For women with eating disorders, the drive to be thin becomes the focal point of their identity, sometimes to the exclusion of all else.

It is important to distinguish between the eating disorders of anorexia nervosa and bulimia. Anorexia is the denial of food to the point of near starvation and resulting weight loss. The anorexic has a distorted body image, often seeing herself as fat even though her weight loss has left her looking emaciated. She typically lives with an intense fear of becoming fat. While it may seem that the anorexic is not interested in food, the opposite is actually true. She may have an incredible amount of nutritional knowledge, which she uses to avoid unnecessary fat or calories in her diet. She may also prepare elaborate meals for others or offer gifts of food, but will not eat these treats herself. The typical anorexic is a high achiever from a good family, who is obedient, over-motivated, and successful academically. Anorexia seems to be a way for the compliant person to react against pressures to be perfect.

Bulimia is an eating disorder that involves episodes of binge eating of high-calorie foods. A person on a binge will consume anywhere from 2,000 calories to 20,000 calories at a time. Afterwards, the bulimic is overcome with guilt and attempts to negate the food she has eaten by purging it. Purging may take the form of vomiting, fasting, use of laxatives or diuretics, or even excessive exercise.

Bulimia is more common than anorexia, and some anorexics may become bulimic over time. According to some experts, 35 percent to 65 percent of college-age women suffer from either anorexia or bulimia. Other, more recent Melpomene studies suggest that this figure is inflated, however. In our 1989 study of 229 college athletes, only 4.7 percent said they had been diagnosed as having an eating disorder. Four percent said they used vomiting as a weight-control method. Overall, it appeared that fewer than 20 percent had problems connected with eating that could be classified as an eating disorder.

There are many psychological and social issues that surround eating disorders, including self-esteem and family expectations. Women who are athletic face additional issues and pressures that may contribute to an eating disorder. For example, women who compete in sports such as running, dance, or gymnastics may believe that they would look better or perform better if they weighed less. Participants in these "thin-body" sports often find themselves involved in unhealthy weight-loss practices; eventually, some of these women may develop an eating disorder.

An athlete's identity can further reinforce this weight-loss cycle. A woman who perceives herself primarily as an athlete may link her self-worth to sports performance. She may feel that she has much to lose if she should gain weight and be unable to do well in her sport. She constantly faces the internal threat: "If I become fat, I will not be an athlete any longer, and if I am not an athlete, then who am I?" Young women who have been in competitive athletics for many years may find the thought of not competing especially frightening, thus reinforcing their struggle to stay thin.

The issue of control can also contribute to eating disorders in athletic women. The high school or collegiate athlete may feel that she has little control over her life, and that her parents, coaches, and teachers are at the helm instead. Chances are she may be striving to do well at all things in order to please the other people in her life. Not eating is a subtle way of exerting control over both herself and others, and may be chosen when the athlete sees no other alternative.

A unique aspect of exercise in relation to eating disorders is that physical activity may be used as a purge. It is not unusual for the woman with an eating disorder to engage in excessive exercise in an attempt to negate food that has been eaten or will be eaten in the future. This purge component of exercise raises interesting questions as we learn more about body image and eating disorders. It is often difficult to tell whether an athlete exercises to become thin or to stay thin, or if that athlete is thin in order to be good at her sport. Even after making that distinction, we still don't know at what point exercise becomes excessive, or when it can be considered part of an eating disorder or purging. These questions are often difficult for coaches or healthcare providers working with athletes to answer.

It seems to us that more research is needed to understand the true size and scope of the problem as well as how to treat it best. One of the problems is in identifying women with distorted eating habits. A bulimic, for instance, will hide her eating habits, making it hard to offer her help at the early stages. Once the problem surfaces, friends, family, and coaches are often poorly equipped to help her find treatment. Thankfully, because of the publicity about eating disorders in the last few years, there are now more seminars and books available on how to identify and help eating-disordered women. National organizations that provide this sort of information are listed in the Bibliography.

Because of the increased media coverage relating to eating disorders, many coaches say they are careful when talking to their athletes about weight loss. Coaches are in a unique position to influence young athletes, both as role models and as sources of guidance. A coach's insensitive comment can be damaging, especially if it plays into the doubts and misperceptions that many athletes have about their bodies. As one athlete states, "At age fourteen, my cycling coach told me I was 'fat' in front of my entire team . . . At 5'5", 124 pounds, I was not fat, but my self-esteem was so low that I simply believed him. After all, he was the coach." Comments like this one often incite a round of weight-loss attempts that may someday develop into an eating disorder. Being aware of this possibility is essential for anyone who works with active young women. These days, we are inundated with requests from coaches, trainers, and athletes asking for information about better nutrition, not weight loss. Instead of urging their athletes to eat less, coaches try to focus on eating smarter. We think it's a healthy trend.

CHANGING YOUR ATTITUDE TOWARD FOOD

Although there are hundreds of books and articles on eating and dieting, most of us do not have accurate information about food choices. Studies that measure how much we actually know about calorie content in foods, for instance, suggest that our estimates are frequently inaccurate. Sonia Blackman, Timothy Mertz, and Robert Singer, associates with the Center for Social and Behavioral Science Research at the University of California, asked fifty-three men and eighty-two women whose average age was twenty-four to estimate calories in various foods. Most people were accurate when estimating the number of calories in main meals, but were way off-base when it came to desserts and snacks. They were much more likely to think that desserts were more caloric than main entrees.

How do you compare? Are you likely to skip dessert but have a small second helping of a casserole or salad with dressing? You may be surprised to learn that the dessert you are longing for may have fewer calories than the stroganoff you took instead. If you're one of those people for whom dinner is not complete without dessert, you may be better off eating less of the main course and "saving" some calories for dessert. As Alice, one of our members, says, "It doesn't make any sense for me to totally cut out desserts. I know that I'll end up eating something sweet before I go to bed."

For Alice, enjoying her dessert is a wise decision. Many women prob-

Conference Participant's Ratings of Foods

	Good	*Bad*	*Neutral*
Cheese (1-inch cube)	21	1	14
Yogurt (1 cup)	28	—	8
Pancakes (1 cake)	12	4	19
Milk (skim, 1 cup)	32	1	3
Beer (12 oz)	7	16	13
Bread	31	2	3

Source: Melpomene research participants from LaCrosse, Wisconsin, conference, October 1987.

Current nutritional theories have apparently had an impact on this well-educated group because bread, broiled chicken, and milk are all chosen as "good" foods by the majority of respondents. Next compare the ratings you selected with the following chart that indicates calories and nutrient content. While some of the foods most people mark as "bad" may be high in calories, they may also have good nutrient value. If you also called these foods "bad," it may be time to reeducate yourself. In the process, you'll probably discover that some of the "bad" foods that you love can be included in your normal diet. In moderation, none of the foods listed are truly *bad!*

Calories and Nutrients of Selected Foods

Foods	*Calories*	*Main Nutrients*
Chicken, broiled (3 oz)	115	Prot, Ca, P, K, Vit A
Eggs, hard boiled (one)	80	Prot, Fat, Ca, P, K, Vit A, SF acid
Sirloin steak (3 oz)	220	Prot, Fat, SF acid, Oleic acid, Ca, P, K
Fish, deep fried (3 oz)	140	Prot, Ca, P, K, Fat
Ice cream (1 cup 10 percent fat)	255	Carbo, Fat, SF acid, Ca, Vit A, Prot
Potato chips (10 medium)	115	Carbo, Ca, K, Na, Vit C, Fat
Popcorn (1 cup with oil and salt)	40	Carbo
Cheese (1-inch cube)	70	Prot, Ca, Vit A, Fat
Yogurt (1 cup)	125	Carbo, Prot, Fat, Ca, P, Vit A
Pancakes (1 cake)	60	Carbo, Ca, Vit A

Calories and Nutrients of Selected Foods

Foods	*Calories*	*Main Nutrients*
Milk (skim, 1 cup)	90	Carbo, Prot, Ca
Beer (12 oz)	150	Carbo, Ca, Niacin
Bread (whole wheat, 1 slice)	65	Carbo, Prot, Ca
Bread (white, 1 slice)	70	Carbo, Prot, Ca

KEY: Prot = protein, Ca = calcium, P = phosporus, K = Potassium, SF acid = saturated fatty acid, Carbo = carbohydrates, Na = Sodium, Vit A = vitamin A.
Source: Nutritive Value of Food, 1982 United States Department of Agriculture, Home and Garden Bulletin, #72.

Changing your own attitudes about food will make you more aware of how many people are overly concerned with food choices. Try this experiment. The next time you eat with friends or relatives make a mental note of how many people talk about what they should or should not be eating. How many people say that they are "bad" if they consider a piece of pie or a second slice of bread? What do you think this kind of labeling does to self-esteem?

Many of us judge what we should or shouldn't eat by our most current reading on the scale. When taken to the extreme, weight scales can become instruments of torture. In the past five years, another method of gauging fitness or obesity has become popular. As you will see below, there are many different ways of measuring body fat, some more accurate than others. We urge you to find out as much as you can before you get your body fat checked to avoid having this measurement being one more tyrannical number that keeps you from a good, healthy body image.

BODY FAT MEASUREMENTS: MOTIVATOR OR MILLSTONE?

What are body fat measurements? Is it possible to get such a reading at an annual medical checkup? Can you do it yourself? What methods are available and how accurate are they?

Underwater weighing. Some researchers still consider underwater weighing to be the most accurate way to measure body fat. Before taking the measurement, a technician uses a special apparatus to measure your residual oxygen, that is, the oxygen left after you expel all the air from your lungs. You are then lowered into a tank of water on a chair attached to a scale. After recording your underwater weight, the technician raises you from the water and then repeats the procedure about six times to assure accurate measurement. Because people's bone mineral content and body water vary, this method leads to an overestimation of body fat in older women and an underestimation in an athletic population. The method is also somewhat tedious and requires sophisticated equipment and skilled technicians.

Skinfold. Research has also validated the usefulness of skinfold measurement to determine body fat. In this method, the technician uses a caliper to measure the thickness of pinched skin at specified points on the body. Generalized equations for predicting body density were developed by researchers Jackson and Pollock and described in the *British Journal of Nutrition* in 1978. These equations have become accepted and are widely used by the Y's and other fitness centers.

Computer testing. Within the last five years, a third method of measuring body fat has also become available. This method, known as the electrical impedance method, is based on how much fluid the cells contain and how quickly an electrical charge can move through them. Electricity moves fastest through fat-free cells because they are primarily made up of fluid, whereas fat cells have only 14 percent of this conducting medium. To take the measurement, a technician hooks up electrodes to your body and introduces a low-voltage charge. As the charge travels through your body, it is slowed down by the fat compartments, but moves freely through the fat-free cells. By analyzing how easily the charge passes through your cells, the device can estimate how much of your body is made up of fat.

Karen Husu, clinical nutrition manager at United and Children's Hospitals in St. Paul, Minnesota, currently uses this method to assess body fats on a monthly basis for YMCA members, for hospital employees, and for clients receiving counseling for weight control. This method relies on accurate knowledge or measurement of body weight, height, and age—all factors in the formula used to derive the percentage of body fat. The success of this method, like the other two described, depends on how careful and experienced the operator is. Husu has used the method for two years and reports that it is not accurate for the very obese or for the competitive athlete. Also, because fluid is so important in the test, she has found that dehydration can cause errors.

WHICH METHOD IS BEST?

With all the possibilities for error, is it worth trying to get your body fat measured? What is the best method? Melpomene Institute has conducted research using both underwater weighing and skinfold measurements. Our findings suggest that accurate caliper measurement can be effectively used in the research setting. We've also seen evidence that as long as health professionals and physical educators are adequately trained, they can take accurate skinfold readings at hospitals and health clubs. Since it is also considerably faster and more economical than underwater weighing, skinfold measurement is our method of choice. We urge you to be wary, however, of the inexpensive calipers advertised in fitness magazines. Most are not useful at all; they are poorly calibrated, and, since some practice is needed for accuracy, it is difficult to perform the test on yourself or on friends. Your best bet is to be measured by a professional and, if you want to recheck your measurements at a later date, try to have it done by the same person or at the same facility.

A warning: If you are like many women who experience a two- to five-pound water-weight gain just before their period, your body fat percentage may also be influenced by the stage of your menstrual cycle. Diane Wakat, Ph.D., professor and nutritional counselor at the University of Virginia, finds that specific site measurements might vary by as much as 3 mm on certain days, resulting in a body fat that fluctuates by 3 percent to 5 percent. According to Wakat, most women can expect their body fat to be highest during the four to six days before their period. Coaches who set specific body fat limits for their athletes (e.g., below 18 percent) don't always recognize the fact that a woman may measure 18 percent one week and 23 percent the next. The water weight that causes the fluctuation will also affect girth measurements and computerized methods of determining body fat.

Well, you may be thinking, it sounds as if all methods have margins of error; it doesn't seem as if any of these readings are absolute. Why not just continue to evaluate myself by how much I weigh? What if I discover my body fat percentage is "worse" than my weight?

Even though the measurement of body fat has some problems, it is a better way to measure fitness than by scale weight. Weight as measured on a scale says little about the composition of that weight. Since muscle weighs more than fat, a muscular person will weight more on a scale. A well-toned, muscled body, however, looks better and burns calories more efficiently than a flabby body. Look at yourself in the mirror. The way you look depends in large part on your fitness. It always surprises women to learn that someone who weighs 145 pounds can have only 19 percent body fat. On the other hand, sedentary women who may have believed they were a good weight may find their body fat to be higher than they would like it to be.

The problem is that we have all been socialized to have some idea of what "fat" is on a scale and so are apt to judge our own body image on that basis. Body fat percentages are new to us, and we don't yet know what a "good" body fat percentage would be for our age, height, and weight. To begin, you'll need some idea of the range of body fats in both active and sedentary populations.

PUTTING BODY FAT PERCENTAGES IN PERSPECTIVE

To avoid letting body fat measurements become another unreachable goal, it's important for you to know that "normal" body fat for nonathletic women is 28 percent to 30 percent. A figure of 22 percent to 25 percent represents fitness and relative slimness. Covert Bailey, who publishes a newsletter on body fat issues, wrote the following in December 1982:

> Adult women below 22 percent body fat are rare. I see plenty of them because our program attracts healthy athletic people, but they represent a small fraction of the population. There are only a few body fat studies on very young children, but the evidence is that pre-puberty girls [who] are normally active stay below 15 percent body fat. After puberty, female fat levels tend to rise, and rise, and rise, stopping at a healthy 22

percent only for those who exercise regularly. It seems that approximately 22 percent fat is a natural and healthy percent fat for women with normal female hormone levels and moderate *playtime* exercise programs. To stay below 22 percent seems to require special attention to exercise and diet.

Bailey, who has measured the body fats of many athletic women using the underwater weighing method, finds that a woman needs to be "professionally involved" with exercise to achieve the 18 percent level desired by many. Aerobic dance instructors and women who regularly compete as runners or triathletes are more likely to achieve these levels, he says, but even they usually modify their diets to maintain the weight.

Unfortunately, Bailey's information is not common knowledge. In our research with physically active women, we are finding that women would prefer to have a somewhat lower percentage of body fat than what is considered average. This preference was highlighted by a 1982 Melpomene study conducted with low-mileage runners who said they really wanted to measure 19 percent body fat, which is lower than the average, active woman's range of 22 percent to 25 percent. Even more damaging was the fact that many of these women were comparing themselves with the few, elite distance runners they had read about who average 13 percent body fat. As long as they were exercising, the women felt that they should be able to achieve a 15 percent or lower body fat reading, which is nearly half of what they might realistically be.

When the Melpomene staff measured body fats at a women's YWCA race in 1985, we heard firsthand how important these measurements were becoming to women. The lines were long, as they usually are when body fat testing is offered. The women who waited were a diverse group, ranging from very fast, nationally ranked runners to women who had never in their lives run 6.2 miles. Their conversations with one another underscored the need for better education about body fat. "Body fat is a better measure of fitness," said one, "so I plan to put more importance on this reading than on my scale weight." Another said, "I'm hoping that my body fat measurement will finally tell me I'm not overweight, or at least not overfat. If my body fat reading is 16 percent then I can stop worrying."

How do you react to these statements? At Melpomene, we're concerned. Too many women spend their lives searching for an outside, objective source that will tell them that their body is okay. As long as their internal self-confidence and body image remain low, we believe that even a "good" reading won't stop the search. In many cases, physically active women know they look and feel better because of their activity, and yet they still worry.

So what if you measure 16 percent body fat? If it will indeed stop you from fixating on food or on being fat, then it may have some merit. But what if you measure 17 percent or 18 percent? If you know yourself well enough to know that any body fat will be discouraging, you are like the many women who stand cautiously in line and question us thoroughly before we begin the simple measurements. Some back out. "I don't need another discouraging measure!" is a typical comment.

At the 1985 race we remeasured fifteen or twenty women who had recently had their body fats measured by the electrical impedance method at local health clubs. Our measurements were consistently five percentage points lower than a reading taken within the last month with the alternate method. "Oh, that's great! Thank you. Is this method really accurate?" asked these women. We quickly gathered a group of women who wanted to know more about the different methods. From their stories we learned how devastating the results of a high body fat reading can be. Even though the higher reading caused distress, many were ready to accept the electrical impedance figure; they believed it to be highly accurate because it involved electrodes and a computer!

Kay, laughingly but with some embarrassment, shared the fact that after a year of exercise she had become much happier with her body:

> I had lost very little weight on the scale but my clothes fit differently. One of my sons said he really liked the muscles on my legs. I felt pretty good and thought that I would verify the changes with a body fat measurement. The club measured me at 28 percent! Since I had just been reading my first runner's magazine about women who were 13 percent body fat, I was really discouraged. To be honest, I went out and bought a fad diet book. I've been following that diet for three weeks now and the only results I see are that I'm crabbier, harder to live with, and my running is worse. I don't have the energy.

When we measured Kay at 23 percent body fat, she was ecstatic and skeptical. "I'd love to believe this evaluation," she said, "but how can it be accurate?" After comparing methods and describing some of the pos-sibilities for error in each method, I think we convinced her that her true body fat was closer to 23 percent than 28 percent. Finally, we reminded all the women that while body fat measurements can be used as a fitness indicator, they can also be misused. Using the new numbers as evidence that you are not meeting some false, external standard can be self-defeating. Instead, we recommend that you look for realistic changes in body fat, and use them to pat yourself on the back for your wise decision to start exercising.

DOES EXERCISE MAKE A DIFFERENCE?

Becoming physically active can change your body shape by toning and hardening your muscles and lowering your body fat over time. It may not mean that you weigh less on the scale, however. In fact, since muscle weighs more than fat, some women's weight may increase slightly with exercise. Lyle is a good example. When she started exercising, she was not overweight, but she was overfat. Three weeks after she began running and weight training, she noticed that her clothes fit more loosely around her waist. After six weeks, friends and colleagues remarked on her changed body. Expecting to find a major drop in weight, Lyle was dis-mayed to find that the scale reading had crept up. Exercise had burned the fat, but it built up muscle, causing her scale weight to climb. For-tunately, the positive comments Lyle received convinced her that she was moving in the right direction and did not need to be dismayed by her weight gain.

Lyle's experience is not the norm, however. If you are like most women, you can expect to lose some weight after taking up a regular exercise program. You should probably not expect to lose more than five to fifteen pounds in a year, however. At first this change will occur with-out major changes to your diet. As you become more skilled or perhaps competitive in your activity, you may want to drop more weight. In our studies, we found that women runners were still concerned with weight, even after they had become wonderfully fit. This concern seems to stem from the notion that being thinner will improve performance. Although this belief has never been proven conclusively, the antidotal "evidence" has made it a powerful myth. Women who become competitive quickly learn that if someone says, "You're looking good," they mean that you have lost several pounds.

Once you pass the level of change that occurs naturally with exercise, it may be harder to shave off those extra few pounds. You'll have to change your diet if you want to lose more weight. Many physically active women are able to modify their diets without professional help by concentrating on the nutrient value of what they are eating instead of counting calories. Some of these shifts seem to happen almost naturally. "I used to eat red meat on a daily basis," said Carla, "but after three or four months of running, it just didn't taste good anymore." "High fat or protein diets really make me sluggish," say others.

Women who become serious about physical activity tend to find new friends who are also living active lives. Not surprisingly, food is often the topic of conversation. Members of the Northern Lights running club, founded in 1977 by a group of women in the Minneapolis/St. Paul area, have a tradition of eating together after they run. The food at one of their typical Saturday morning brunches is tempting and nutritious. Recipe ideas are exchanged at the meeting and there is discussion about what foods might provide the most energy with the fewest calories. New books on diet and the athlete are discussed, and since most of these women do not have time to develop elaborate new menus or weight the merits of the latest vegetarian diet, they share information about food that seems practical.

Unfortunately, exercise is not a panacea, and all women who are physically active do not come to peaceably accept their bodies. Ellen, age fifty-six, is a good example of someone who exercises regularly, yet still worries excessively about her weight and food intake. An avid hiker, she began walking regularly, at least three miles a day, when she was fifty-two. Ellen grew up on a farm where physical activity was expected and often required. She ate balanced meals, and though she was never thin, she remained a healthy 27 percent body fat until she was forty-nine. While going through menopause, she noticed that she was gaining weight although her diet remained the same. Cutting down on calories didn't seem to help. At the same time, Ellen realized that the stress of her job seemed to be causing headaches and backaches. A friend encouraged her to go walking as part of an informal Saturday morning group. Skeptical at first, Ellen soon found that she loved the exercise and was meeting new women with whom she could share thoughts and concerns. In the first six months, she not only had fewer headaches and backaches but also noticed a difference in how clothes fit and how she looked.

Two years later, Ellen found that her body had learned to use calories more efficiently so that exercise was not enough. She decided she needed to limit calories in order to maintain a body fat that she felt was acceptable. Ellen began to agonize over the calories of everything she ate. Eventually she began to avoid social situations involving food.

The problem of distorted body image had more severe consequences for Beth. Beth started running in her late twenties. Her goal was twofold: to lose some weight and to become a competent runner. She had several running friends whom she admired for their thin bodies and their strength. Beth achieved her goal of competence in the first two years of running. She often placed in her age category in local races and continually improved her times. Initially she also experienced some weight loss as a result of running and changed her diet. But Beth also loved to eat and had certain food desires that she found impossible to curb. She eventually become bulimic, eating vast quantities of cookies, ice cream, and crackers in binges that she hid from her closest friends.

These reactions, fortunately, are exceptions rather than the rule. For most women, taking up exercise helps them to put less importance on the issue of weight. Women participating in another Melpomene study indicate that physical activity often improves overall body image and self-esteem. Some women talk about a changed attitude toward calories. "I'm proud to say that my attitudes about myself and food have been shifting; I realize that I paid too much attention to food and calories in the past . . . I really don't think in terms of calories very much anymore. I've become more concerned with good nutrition."

Others have begun to look at their bodies in new ways. Some talk about new perceptions. "I've decided to appreciate my curves and have decided they are womanly rather than fat!" Others talk about the function of their bodies:

"Running puts me in touch with my body, how it functions and feels under different situations."

"I feel stronger and more fit. I like looking more muscular instead of flabby."

"I like finding out that my body can do things it couldn't do before."

"I feel very positive; I feel strong and appreciate how my body looks."

"My body feels like it is me, and if I like myself, which I do, I have to like my body, too."

The women making these remarks ranged in weight from two hundred to three hundred and fifty pounds. As participants at a 1989 Melpomene conference for larger women entitled "Enhancing Body Image, Fitness, and Health," they were affirming the fact that one can be large and healthy.

BODY IMAGE AND SELF-ESTEEM

Surprisingly, the way we feel about our bodies does not always correlate with how we feel about our self-worth or self-esteem. Psychologists have found that we can have a good body image and low self-esteem or vice versa. Body image is only one of the factors that contributes to self-esteem; there are many other contributing factors. Sometimes, a good body image is not enough to boost self-esteem above the threshold of worthiness.

Consider Jane, for example, who had a body that men admired, and therefore she never worried or even thought much about food. Jane grew up in a home where good eating habits were established early; the meals were well-balanced, low in fat and protein, and high in complex carbohydrates. When Jane was in junior high school, some of her friends remarked on the lack of junk food in her house; Jane confessed that she envied them and loved to come to their homes to "gorp out." For the most part, however, Jane found no reason to change the way she ate.

When many of her friends were becoming heavier and very concerned about body appearance and fat, Jane grew tall and wondered why everyone else spent so much time worrying about food. Her good body, however, did not insulate Jane from other problems. She was not a good student and constantly fought to get good grades. She had difficulty getting along with an older sister who envied Jane's slim-without-a-struggle body. She had few friends, and began to blame her good body for her loneliness, even though the issues were clearly more complex. By the end of her first year in college, Jane's outward appearance fooled many people who could not believe that her self-image was so vulnerable.

By the same token, a bad body image will not necessarily drag down a buoyant self-esteem. Consider Eva, who did not have the perfect body. Even her youngest baby pictures showed someone who was decidedly fat. Some of her earliest memories include being called "Fats" in kindergarten and being chosen last for the teams at recess. It seemed to her that people spent far too much time assessing her body instead of her talents. She could, after all, bat better than most boys, and her sturdy body was often an asset in touch football. Eva also enjoyed books, photography, and school. She spent a lot of time reading, and for several years had few friends because she was not only fat but also a good student. Eva learned to downplay grades without ever giving up her love of learning or her drive to succeed. In high school, she discovered she had acting talent and began to acquire friends and self-confidence. Even though she dieted constantly and was clearly dissatisfied with her body image, her self-esteem was still far better than Jane's.

If you see yourself in either Jane or Eva's stories, take heart. Body image and self-esteem are both dynamic processes that can evolve and change throughout your life. A low time in your life doesn't have to last forever. Shedding the self-consciousness and shame of a poor body image can give you the courage to work on other parts of your life such as self-esteem. Remember: It's never too late to start loving your body.

BODY IMAGE AND AGE

Having positive feelings about your body is a definite advantage as you grow older and begin to encounter the unique image problems related to aging. In a society where the model of feminine beauty is a teenage movie star, older women are in a losing battle. One of the more impossible expectations is that women will remain the same weight throughout life. One Melpomene study asking what weight was "just right" for a 5′4″ woman found that 113 pounds was selected for those under age nineteen and 120–122 pounds for anyone older. This choice is unrealistic and unhealthy for most older women.

The problem for older women may be a lack of positive depictions of women in their age group. As Martha, a striking, gray-haired woman in our osteoporosis study remarked, "I have a problem. I don't have any real role models for how I should look or behave." To put yourself in Martha's place, think about the media images that flash before you every day; most images are of women under forty. Older women are either invisible or are unbelievably glamorous women like Elizabeth Taylor, Lena Horne, and Joan Collins. The television show, "The Golden Girls," is one of the few series where perfect body shape and no wrinkles are not requirements. Interestingly, the show has received excellent ratings and may be indicating how eager older women are for positive reflections of themselves.

As a whole, we don't have much research information that tracks how older women see their bodies. In a current review of all the literature on body image, only six studies included older adults in the sample. Melpomene's studies of older women are among the only sources to which we can turn. Our studies indicate that overall, satisfaction with looks increases with age. In our 1985 study, 39 percent of women ages twenty to twenty-nine believed they looked better than most women, while 87 percent of women over fifty chose that response.

Physical activity seems to boost that positive response even higher. In a follow-up body image questionnaire answered by women in the Melpomene osteoporosis study (see page 177), 96 percent of the high-activity group were generally satisfied with the way they look; this was also true of 76 percent of the medium-activity group and 72 percent of the low-activity group. Sixty-seven percent of the high-activity group were *quite* satisfied, which was twice as many as the low-activity group.

Not only does physical activity favorably influence body image but it also seems to have an impact on health. Sixty-three percent of the high-activity group stated that their health was much better than most, while only 7 percent of the women with a low-activity rating chose that response. Ninety-eight percent of the high-activity group said they had a feeling of looking strong and healthy as compared with 85 percent of the medium-activity group and 57 percent of the low-activity group.

In many ways, it is a shame that we don't start feeling better about our bodies at an earlier age. Some of the older women we spoke to regretted that they had spent so much time, energy, and money chasing after an idealized version of beauty instead of just celebrating the body they had. As we have seen, our society perpetuates the myth that a woman needs to improve herself because she is, presumably, imperfect in some way. Convincing yourself otherwise is a great challenge, but it's worth it.

BECOMING COMFORTABLE WITH THE BODY YOU HAVE

How can you begin to like your body better? The following case studies may give you some ideas for possible changes. Age need not be a barrier. Gwen began to cross-country ski when she was sixty-three. She had almost abandoned exercise after years of physical activity related both to her job as a part-time physical education instructor and family hiking and biking trips. Subtle changes in both body shape and appetite encouraged her to try something new. "As a kid," she recalled, "I was always active in team sports. It was rare, but I attended a private school where those opportunities were available. I guess I always saw myself as fairly skilled athletically and it helped me deal with being 5'11". I also thought that because of my height I would never get fat and out of shape." She laughed. "I have some pictures to show that wasn't true in my later years. I love skiing," she said, "because it has made me fit again, but most importantly, it's given me a sense of independence and strength."

Because she had been a fat child, Jenny still thought of herself as fat even when she had become an almost skinny adult. Competitive running did little to improve her body image. She continued to carefully watch what she ate and rarely consumed more than 1,000 calories per day. After several years of running, her weight stabilized at 105 pounds. Her efficient body seemed to know when she ate more and she frequently noted a 3-pound weight gain after a weekend of heavier eating. Following an injury, Jenny found that her weight began to creep up. Since she thought it unhealthy to eat fewer than 1,000 calories, she began to accept herself at a higher weight. Jenny is now 10 pounds heavier; it still bothers her when she sees how sleek some of her running friends remain. She still struggles with wishing she could eat more, but has learned to accept her new body shape. For the first time when she looks at old pictures she actually thinks she was too thin. But her new perceptions remain vulnerable and she still needs to be reassured that she really doesn't look fat.

Gwen's and Jenny's stories suggest that change will probably be easier if your body image was positive as a child. It may encourage you to pay attention to your own children's attitudes and perceptions. If you have some concerns about your body image, now might be a good time to try to put these concerns into perspective. Once you have done that, change will be easier.

TAKE OBJECTIVE MEASUREMENTS

First, think about how you perceive your body—large, skinny, average, and so on. Then compare your perceptions to actual measurements. If weight is a major issue for you, put yourself on a scale (many women hide from scales) and compare your weight to the table of average-weight ranges for your age and body frame. Next, call your local Y, health club, or clinic to see if they offer body fat testing. If your body fat is within the healthy range, you may be more fit than you think! There is a lot of misinformation floating around about body fat. Keep in mind, however, that the healthy range for body fat may be far broader than either the media or the medical profession would have us believe.

Next, look at pictures of yourself; group pictures may be especially useful. Subconsciously, you may have already ranked yourself in size and weight against the rest of your friends and colleagues. Take a good look now at the evidence; are you really fatter than the rest of the group or is this feeling part of a perception problem?

With whom do you usually compare yourself? Is your reference group a fair appraisal of your own fatness and fitness? If you are comparing yourself with television and magazine models, your seventeen-year-old daughter, or competitive athletes, you are clearly stacking the deck. Yet many older women tell us that they continue to worry about that five to ten pounds because they do not have any good comparisons. Many remember their mothers as soft and slightly overweight. "My mother," said Sarah, "was very happy being seen as 'grandmotherly.' She had a very comfortable lap and a wonderful smile. Even though she might have been overweight on a scale, she remained active and healthy until she died at eighty-seven." Sarah wishes that she could feel good about letting her body mellow that way with age. "These days," she says, "a woman is expected to look young and thin until she dies."

CHECK YOUR OWN PERCEPTIONS

Do you have that expectation for yourself and other people? One interesting way to look at body image and decide if you need to work on your own perceptions and goals is to buy a roll of film and take pictures of people of all ages and both sexes. Take your pictures in various public places: a park, a concert, a running race, a baseball game, a shopping center. When you get them developed, look at the expressions on people's faces as well as their external appearance. What kinds of assumptions do you make about these people based on the photos?

Do you find that you are more critical of people who are fat? Are you more critical of fat women than fat men? Earlier, we described some of the myths and negative attitudes that stifle large women. We also showed you evidence that fat women generally do not overeat, and that for some women, being thin will never be a realistic or a healthy option. Even with this new knowledge, you still may be forming judgments based on old stereotypes. One way to test your sensitivity and perhaps reverse your judgments is to take the following test.

F Scale

LISTED BELOW ARE ADJECTIVES SOMETIMES USED TO DESCRIBE OBESE
OR FAT PEOPLE. PLEASE INDICATE YOUR BELIEFS ABOUT WHAT FAT
PEOPLE ARE LIKE ON THE FOLLOWING ITEMS BY PLACING AN *X* ON
THE LINE THAT BEST DESCRIBES YOUR FEELINGS AND BELIEFS.

1. lazy	—— —— —— —— ——	industrious
2. sloppy	—— —— —— —— ——	neat
3. disgusting	—— —— —— —— ——	not disgusting
4. friendly	—— —— —— —— ——	unfriendly
5. nonassertive	—— —— —— —— ——	assertive
6. no willpower	—— —— —— —— ——	has willpower
7. artistic	—— —— —— —— ——	not artistic
8. creative	—— —— —— —— ——	uncreative
9. warm	—— —— —— —— ——	cold
10. depressed	—— —— —— —— ——	happy
11. smart	—— —— —— —— ——	stupid
12. reads a lot	—— —— —— —— ——	doesn't read a lot
13. unambitious	—— —— —— —— ——	ambitious
14. easy to talk to	—— —— —— —— ——	hard to talk to
15. unattractive	—— —— —— —— ——	attractive
16. miserable	—— —— —— —— ——	jolly
17. selfish	—— —— —— —— ——	selfless
18. poor self-control	—— —— —— —— ——	good self-control
19. inconsiderate of others	—— —— —— —— ——	considerate of others
20. good	—— —— —— —— ——	bad
21. popular	—— —— —— —— ——	unpopular
22. important	—— —— —— —— ——	insignificant
23. slow	—— —— —— —— ——	fast
24. ineffective	—— —— —— —— ——	effective
25. careless	—— —— —— —— ——	careful
26. having endurance	—— —— —— —— ——	having no endurance
27. inactive	—— —— —— —— ——	active
28. nice complexion	—— —— —— —— ——	bad complexion

ably unnecessarily limit certain foods because they have mentally classified them as "good" or "bad." Test yourself: Rate the foods on the following list. Do you consider the item "good," "bad," or "neutral" with regard to calories and nutritive value?

My Nutritive Rating of Selected Foods

	Good	Bad	Neutral
Chicken, broiled	❏	❏	❏
Eggs, hard boiled	❏	❏	❏
Sirloin steak	❏	❏	❏
Fish, deep fried	❏	❏	❏
Ice cream	❏	❏	❏
Popcorn	❏	❏	❏
Potato chips	❏	❏	❏
Cheese	❏	❏	❏
Yogurt	❏	❏	❏
Pancakes	❏	❏	❏
Milk	❏	❏	❏
Beer	❏	❏	❏
Bread	❏	❏	❏

This same food test was distributed to participants at a nutrition conference in LaCrosse, Wisconsin, in 1987. See if you agree with their ratings.

Conference Participant's Ratings of Foods

	Good	Bad	Neutral
Chicken, broiled (3 oz)	35	1	—
Eggs, hard boiled (one)	13	8	14
Sirloin steak (3 oz)	11	15	10
Fish, deep fried (3 oz)	—	28	8
Ice cream (1 cup 10 percent fat)	6	17	13

29. tries to please people	—	—	—	—	—	doesn't try to please people
30. humorous/funny	—	—	—	—	—	humorless/not funny
31. inefficient	—	—	—	—	—	efficient
32. strong	—	—	—	—	—	weak
33. individualistic	—	—	—	—	—	not individualistic
34. pitiful	—	—	—	—	—	not pitiful
35. independent	—	—	—	—	—	dependent
36. good-natured	—	—	—	—	—	irritable
37. self-indulgent	—	—	—	—	—	self-sacrificing
38. passive	—	—	—	—	—	aggressive
39. indirect	—	—	—	—	—	direct
40. likes food	—	—	—	—	—	dislikes food
41. dirty	—	—	—	—	—	clean
42. does not attend to own appearance	—	—	—	—	—	very attentive to own appearance
43. easygoing	—	—	—	—	—	uptight
44. shapeless	—	—	—	—	—	shapely
45. overeats	—	—	—	—	—	undereats
46. smells bad	—	—	—	—	—	smells good
47. sweaty	—	—	—	—	—	not sweaty
48. moody	—	—	—	—	—	even-tempered
49. insecure	—	—	—	—	—	secure
50. low self-esteem	—	—	—	—	—	high self-esteem

Source: Developed by B. Robinson in 1984.

Psychologist Beatrice "Bean" Robinson, the author of the 1984 Fat Phobia Scale (F Scale), reports that a majority of the 856 people who filled out her questionnaire chose more negative adjectives than positive ones when asked to describe their feelings and beliefs about fat people. The data show that people do indeed harbor a strong negative stereotype about fat people.

Some of the more common negative comments were that fat people like food, overeat, have low self-esteem, and are insecure, shapeless, and inactive. Respondents also had some positive things to say about fat people, however, commenting that they were friendly, warm, easy to talk to, and humorous.

Robinson administers the Fat Phobia Scale to her fat clients before and after they go through a program created by Robinson and her colleague, psychologist Jane Bacon. The program is designed to improve the self-esteem and body image of obese people who are at least fifty pounds over their recommended weight. The majority of these clients say they have more positive attitudes toward fat people after completing the program, suggesting that fat phobia, which Robinson describes as a fear and hatred of fat people, can be changed by education and group therapy. If you aren't overweight, but are critical of those who are, and fearful of becoming fat yourself, this may be the time to change those attitudes. It may not be easy.

"The *Melpomene Report* article on fat phobia was interesting," remarked a Melpomene volunteer several years ago. "I know I have a prejudice against fat people; I'm always sure they can control their weight!" Having believed that for fifty-eight years, this woman continues to relate stories and experiences that are helping her slowly change her opinions. Fat women are beginning to speak out about their experiences; many are developing self-images that allow them to be secure with who they are. Clothing manufacturers like Beautiful Skier and Fitting Image, and magazines like *Radiance* play a big part in helping these women make that change.

We do not all have the same opportunity to be thin adults. Psychologist Albert Stunkard says that families who have a history of obesity "will really have to work on trying to prevent obesity in their kids." Once these children are adults, they too are going to have to "remain eternally vigilant against gaining weight." Stunkard and his colleagues conclude that the struggle is worth it because of the emotional and physical problems of being overweight.

Do you agree? There are certainly societal disadvantages to being fat. Yet many women, after years of unsuccessful dieting, regret all the time they've wasted worrying about gaining weight. They are eager to explore new ideas and approaches to weight and body image; they want to work on accepting the bodies that they have. Flying in the face of everything society believes about body size, women of all weights are beginning to build foundations of self-respect. Conferences or small groups facilitated by a clinical psychologist are offered in some areas to help women readjust their body images. Some foresighted educators are working with young women before the lifetime patterns of self-loathing become too deeply ingrained.

An ideal time to work on these concepts is in high school or college. Leslie McBride, a professor in the school of health and physical education at Portland State University, has worked with adolescents in a group situation designed to get them to look more objectively and positively at themselves. She asks them to make two lists: One enumerates positive physical features about one's self, and the other lists negative features. Next, cards with the names of each participant are distributed. The group is then instructed to write down a positive comment about the physical appearance of the person whose name appears on the top of the card.

Imagine the results. Many students reported that they had never really thought about themselves as they were described by others. Being told that you have particularly beautiful eyes, that you look strong, or that your smile always encourages others has a positive influence that can affect the way you feel about your body.

A similar exercise would be a good starting place for adults trying to work on body image issues. Try a simple test. Ask any friend about her best physical features; she will probably hesitate at first and often not even be aware of something that others find particularly attractive or outstanding.

Janette's hair started to turn gray long before many of her friends. After several years of fooling around with coloring, she decided it wasn't worth the effort. Suddenly people started complimenting her on her beautiful hair, which to this day surprises her. Janette's experience reminds us that the image we have of ourselves may be worlds different than how others see us. Learning to accept and believe genuine compliments may help you start to change your inner picture of yourself.

GET MOVING

Being or becoming physically active is a great way to improve your body image and boost your confidence in other areas as well. Don't be discouraged if early attempts to play tennis, walk, or run are not an immediate success. Having a body that functions well will definitely increase self-esteem. Functioning will, however, have different meanings for different ages, shapes, and abilities. Naturally, the woman who is sixty and has arthritis will not be able to do the same things as the sixteen-year-old gymnast. The twenty-five-year-old athlete who has become quadriplegic as the result of an accident will also have to modify her perspective of what it means to be physically active. Yet each of us who begins to see what her body can do will find herself more confident in other areas as well.

KEEP A RECORD OF YOUR PROGRESS

If you have problems in some of the areas discussed in this chapter, begin today to change them! Don't say, "I have to watch what I eat," even though it may take years before you feel differently about your eating habits. Begin to think about things you do well, physically and mentally, and work on those. It may help to make a list of things you like about yourself, again both physical and mental qualities, and put it somewhere where you can read it six months later. One of the best ways to keep track of your feelings and progress is to start a diary.

Edith bought a slender, lined book when she was thirty-seven. She had been having problems at work, her relationship with her spouse of fifteen years showed signs of strain, and she wasn't sure what was happening. She had read that keeping a journal might be helpful and decided to try to write whenever she was moved to do so. Now, twelve years later, Edith has eight volumes of thoughts and musings. While she is not sure they have ever been responsible for solving major problems, the act of writing things down has often been helpful. About once a year, she takes the time to skim through her journals to see if she can find anything useful or revealing. She is encouraged by the fact that she seems more mellow and is certainly happier with her body (although it's enlarging and slipping downward).

For Edith keeping a personal journal was enough; the act of writing helped her express anger and joy. It helped articulate problems and identify options. Over the years, rereading the journal has been both instructive and soothing.

FIND PEOPLE WHO WILL NURTURE YOU

Samantha, in contrast, doesn't express herself well in writing. She found that talking to her friends was the best way for her to sort through her body and self-image problems. As a runner who was returning to school as a much older student, she had numerous concerns about fitting in and being successful. One thing that helped her work through these issues was to start a running group with other women who were in the same situation. "I found that the act of running made me more open in my remarks; as my friendship with that small group of women developed, I was able to discuss things I never would have thought possible."

Other women may wish or need to seek professional advice and help. While some of the good weight-loss programs also deal with issues of self-esteem and change, they usually connect these improvements with becoming thinner. When this is not your objective, it may be more difficult to find a psychologist, nutritionist, or physician who will be sympathetic and knowledgeable about your concerns.

The following suggestions may help you select the appropriate professional. If possible, find someone who has experience with clients who have body image concerns or problems. It may be worthwhile to talk with one of the clients to gain a better understanding of the professional's perspective and usual methods. Some believe that a change in behaviors leads to a change in attitudes. Others prefer to move from attitudes toward changed behaviors. Still others, who have a more flexible style, will move in whatever direction works for you.

Once you have identified several nutritionists or psychologists, the next step is to talk with one or two of them on the phone. Look for someone who treats you seriously. Ann Meissner, a psychologist who has been a speaker at numerous Melpomene conferences, suggests that you conduct an interview on the phone, or perhaps in person. This first conversation should do more than answer questions about the process; you should also come away with the feeling that the professional likes you and is willing to help you work through your issues. Meissner also says that she seldom recommends that a client see a therapist who is younger. A certain amount of empathy will come from having experienced some things firsthand.

A good professional should be able to help you start accepting your body.

If weight loss is part of a sensible program, be sure that you are getting some psychological support as well. Meissner believes that losing weight can markedly change self-concept. In fact, it occasionally comes as a surprise to many people that this change may have negative as well as positive elements.

Remember that the method the professional prefers may not be a good fit for you. Throughout the process, it will pay for you to evaluate how much progress you feel you are making. If you feel the method is no longer working, perhaps it's time to adjust the approach. Take advantage of the momentum you've already gained to bring you all the way to home base—safe and feeling good inside your own body.

CELEBRATE THE BODY YOU HAVE

Hopefully, after reading this chapter, you have some different perceptions about what constitutes a "good" body. Maybe you would now rank strong and healthy above thin and petite. Maybe you've begun to see your own body more realistically, and begun to appreciate it for its flexibility or muscle tone, rather than haggling over the few extra pounds you've gained this year.

Once you've made friends with your body, you'll need to tend to the relationship as natural changes occur. The flat stomach you are proud of in your twenties will soften and grow rounder with age. Your joints may get stiffer, and your running times may get slower. Or, you could become disabled and not be able to run at all anymore. The challenge is to let your standards change along with your body and to congratulate yourself for who you are at that particular moment.

It's a wonderful feeling to be proud of your body. Gaining physical confidence can alter the way you see yourself in the world. For Diana Nyad, the swimmer, being a physically strong woman makes her feel like "she owns the earth." At Melpomene, we like to try to imagine what the world would be like if we all ignored the cultural prescriptions for female beauty and began to feel at home in our own bodies. Think of what we could do with all the time and energy we currently spend dieting and "improving" ourselves!

T H R E E
MENSTRUAL FACT AND FICTION

Susan, age eighteen, has been running since she was twelve. During the winter she competes on her school's cross-country skiing team, and in the warm months she runs as much as forty miles in a week. Susan has never had a menstrual period, and both she and her mother are concerned. Susan is worried because her body has not shown many characteristics of puberty. Her mother is concerned that Susan is not "normal," and has urged her daughter to seek medical advice.

Danielle started exercising five years ago. During the warm weather, she walks or bikes four or five days a week, and in the winter she swims. Danielle noticed that her menstrual periods changed once she became physically active. Cramps were fewer and the flow seemed lighter. Although these changes were inconsequential, Danielle wondered if they were related to her exercise program.

Cynthia, age twenty-nine, began running seven years ago. She became serious about the sport when she discovered that she had talent as a runner. Cynthia's training program often includes mileage of forty to fifty miles per week. As a result of diet change and the high mileage, she has lost about ten pounds. Cynthia stopped having menstrual periods three years ago and is concerned about her health. She wonders if the absence of periods is unhealthy and if she will ever be able to have children.

WHAT IS NORMAL?

Most women have concerns from time to time about their menstrual cycles and reproductive health. Certainly when there is some noticeable change in our bodies, we tend to wonder if we are "normal." When it comes to menstrual functioning, the term *normal* defies definition and often leaves doctors and researchers baffled. Usually, the average is considered the norm, and if a woman fluctuates far enough away from this average, she may be considered "not normal." We must keep in mind, however, that averages can't describe every case, and what is "not normal" for most women may be perfectly healthy for you.

The average woman experiences menstrual cycles that are anywhere from twenty-four to thirty-two days in length. Most of the time these cycles are ovulatory, which means that an egg is released about midway through the cycle (about fourteen days before bleeding starts). Not every menstrual cycle is ovulatory, however. Occasionally, a cycle may be anovulatory—one in which an egg is not released.

Hormones of various kinds have major roles in the menstrual cycle. Two of the most prominent are estrogen and progesterone. Estrogen is the key player from day one (when bleeding starts) through day fourteen of the cycle. Throughout this *follicular phase*, estrogen is rising and the uterine lining or endometrium is building up, preparing for ovulation and possible pregnancy. Estrogen levels peak just before ovulation, then drop dramatically.

As estrogen is starting to rise during the first week of the cycle, another hormone called follicle stimulating hormone (FSH) is released by the pituitary gland. FSH, which causes the growth and maturation of ovarian follicles in preparation for ovulation, is at a slightly elevated level during the first week and then drops off again until about day fourteen. When ovulation is about to occur, FSH, and a fourth hormone called luteinizing hormone (LH), both rise to peak levels that cause a now mature follicle to release the egg.

For the next two weeks of the cycle, or the *luteal phase*, there is a rise in progesterone, a hormone that "ripens" the endometrium. As progesterone decreases toward the end of this luteal phase, and if no pregnancy has occurred, bleeding will begin, and the menstrual flow will last about four to seven days. The figure below illustrates hormonal levels during the menstrual cycle.

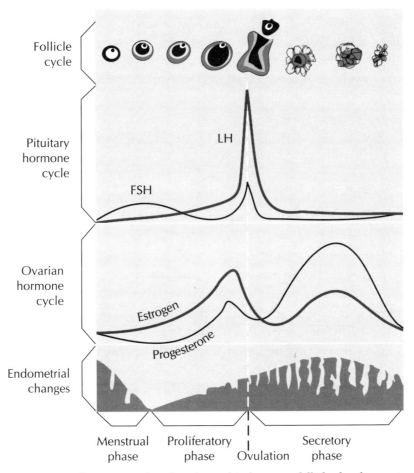

Figure 3.1: The menstrual cycle relationship between follicle development, hormone cycles, and endometrial (uterine lining) buildup and disintegration. The cervical mucus gets progressively wetter from the menstrual phase to ovulation, then becomes drier during the secretory phase.

Source: Reprinted with permission from the Boston Women's Health Book Collective: *The New Our Bodies Ourselves,* by Peggy Clark, Simon and Schuster: New York, 1984.

Again, not all women fit this average profile, and variations do not mean that their health is in danger. Rather, they may be experiencing wider fluctuations within what is still considered the normal and healthy range. For example, while the interval between ovulation and menstrual flow is usually constant at fourteen days, the preovulatory period from menstruation to ovulation may vary from seven to thirty days or more in some women, which explains why menstrual cycles sometimes vary in length.

A number of factors can affect the menstrual timing and flow, including diet, stress, weight loss, or physical activity. In this chapter, we will look at how your exercise program may or may not impact your menstrual cycle, and what changes you might expect over time.

MINOR MENSTRUAL CYCLE CHANGES AND EXERCISE

DYSMENORRHEA

"I feel better if I can get myself to exercise; I'm less depressed."

"I often need to curtail my physical activity during the first days of my period due to increased flow and cramping."

"Throughout high school and the first two years of college, I was almost bedridden with severe cramping, nausea, vomiting, and heavy bleeding due to my period. I missed school and was on medication."

"The only change that occurred was in the first one or two years after I began to run on a year-round basis. My mileage went from twenty or thirty to forty or fifty per week. My periods became lighter and less frequent for about a year and a half, until my body adjusted and my periods went back to 'normal.' "

"I notice my cramping more when I'm running or swimming. It seems more intense."

Remember your high school gym teacher telling you that physical activity was the best way to alleviate menstrual discomfort? Research is showing that this belief is not necessarily true; the relationship between menstrual symptoms and physical activity is more complex than we once thought.

A common menstrual complaint is dysmenorrhea, characterized by lower abdominal cramps, which may be accompanied by headache, backache, fatigue, breast soreness, and/or weight gain during the menstrual cycle. Researchers in the 1930s were among the first to recognize dysmenorrhea as physical rather than psychological in origin. Researchers in the past have linked such factors as bad posture, faulty living habits, and the lack of abdominal strength to the occurrence of dysmenorrhea.

Myths surrounding the menstrual period are evident in the following quote from the book *Wife and Mother, or Information for Every Woman*, published by H. J. Smith and Company of Philadelphia in 1888, which states:

> During "the monthly periods," violent exercise is injurious; iced drinks and acid beverages are improper; and bathing in the sea, and bathing the feet in cold water, and cold baths, are dangerous; indeed at such times as these, no risks should be run, and no experiments should, for one moment, be permitted, otherwise serious consequences will, in all probability, ensue. "The monthly periods" are times not to be trifled with, or woe betide the unfortunate trifler! . . . The pale, colorless complexion, helpless, listless, and almost lifeless young ladies, that are so constantly seen in society, usually owe their miserable state of health either to absent, to deficient, or to profuse menstruation. Their breathing is short—they are soon "out of breath"; if they attempt to take exercise—to walk, for instance, either up stairs, or up a hill, or even for half a mile on level ground, their breath is nearly exhausted—they pant as though they had been running quickly. They are ready, after the slightest exertion or fatigue, and after the least worry or excitement, to feel faint, and sometimes even to actually swoon away.

It has been only in the past twenty-five years that researchers have looked at athletic training and its impact on the menstrual cycle. In a 1975 study of 1,435 students, Dr. Allan J. Ryan, editor-in-chief of *The Physician and Sportsmedicine*, concluded that there was little correlation between the severity of dysmenorrhea and levels of physical activity. A study of Olympic athletes in the 1976 Montreal games found that although almost 60 percent of the women reported some change in their menstrual patterns due to intense physical activity, only 12 percent of the women noted a lessening of abdominal cramps. For 6 percent of the women, cramping reportedly increased as a result of their activity.

In 1984, we sent a questionnaire to all Melpomene members to gather information on their general health and lifestyle, and more specifically, to learn something about their menstrual patterns. There were 420 women who answered the questionnaire. The average age was thirty-seven, average weight 130 pounds, and average height 5'5". Admittedly, Melpomene members are probably a more physically active group than the general population. But they do vary in age, type of activity, and level of activity. Very few describe themselves first and foremost as "athletes." The variety within this group offers insights that can't be found in studies of elite female athletes. Even though 90 percent of the women in our study described themselves as in better or much better health than their peers, they did experience a wide variety of menstrual symptoms. The most frequently reported symptoms were monthly weight gain, abdominal cramps, irritability, and change in appetite.

We were not able to detect any relationship between abdominal cramping and physical exercise; those women who were sedentary reported the same frequency of cramping as those who were active. Fluctuations in appetite and mood swings also occurred in both the exercising and the nonexercising groups. We did, however, find some correlation between physical activity and changes in menstrual patterns. Women in the high-activity groups were the ones most likely to report changes such as less frequent menstrual periods, a decrease in the amount of menstrual flow, and a decrease in the number of flow days.

These results suggest new information for the gym teacher of the 1990s. Physical activity, though it may cause lighter or more infrequent periods, will not necessarily "cure" common menstrual symptoms such as cramping, backache, or breast tenderness. The most noticeable effect of physical activity, at least in our study, was seen in menstrual patterns, rather than in the lessening of menstrual discomforts. There are, thankfully, other treatment options for women who suffer from painful menstrual periods. Athletic women, their coaches, and their physicians should be aware of them.

Among the natural ways to alleviate discomfort, diet change and relaxation techniques are often suggested in concert with exercise. There are also several nonprescription remedies on the market, some producing only pain relief, whereas others add a diuretic to lessen water retention. Although these remedies alleviate symptoms in some women, they are not effective for all women or for women with severe symptoms.

For many years, physicians have routinely prescribed narcotics such as codeine or Percodan to relieve cramping and other menstrual symptoms. While these drugs do a great job of combating pain, they also produce troublesome side effects such as sleepiness, light-headedness, and even nausea. For many women, taking narcotic painkillers is just a way of trading one level of dysfunction for another.

Recently, a new family of drugs has entered the scene, bringing many women relief with minimal side effects. These drugs work to inhibit prostaglandins—the substances in your body that cause your uterus, intestines, and other smooth muscles to contract. These contractions produce painful cramps as they squeeze blood from your uterine muscle. Rising levels of prostaglandins are also responsible for the intestinal cramping and diarrhea that many women experience along with menstrual cramps. Prostaglandin-inhibiting drugs block prostaglandin production and activity in the body. These drugs work best if you take them as soon as your flow begins, before your prostaglandin levels are high enough to produce painful cramps. As with any drug, there are side effects and some people are advised not to take them. This includes women with aspirin-induced asthma, gastrointestinal irritation (e.g., peptic ulcer), and anyone who is sensitive to the particular kind of drug prescribed.

Some healthcare providers suggest oral contraceptives, or birth control pills, as a way to relieve severe symptoms. The hormones in oral contraceptives may decrease cramping in several ways. First, they prevent ovulation, and cycles in which no egg is released are usually free from cramping. They also thin the uterine lining and lessen the blood flow, so that uterine contractions are reduced. Last, oral contraceptives probably quiet menstrual cramping by reducing the amount of prostaglandin precursors (substances that have the potential to become prostaglandins) in the endometrium. Though they are known to be effective for some women, oral contraceptives should not generally be used to treat dysmenorrhea unless you also need them for birth control. Before you decide to go on the pill, you'll want to discuss the risks with your doctor, especially if you are over thirty-five, are a smoker, or a concerned with sports performance. (See contraception discussion on page 108.)

While there is no perfect method for relieving menstrual discomfort, symptoms are no longer being ignored or written off as psychological. Menstrual symptoms are recognized as very real, and are receiving well-deserved attention from the medical and scientific community. Another set of changes that affects menstrual patterns may not be as easy to detect as the symptoms we just discussed. Nevertheless, these changes can have significant implications for your health. The following section reviews these major changes, their possible connection to exercise, and the current view of treatment.

MAJOR MENSTRUAL CYCLE CHANGES AND EXERCISE

DELAYED MENARCHE

"Being age nineteen and a half and never having had a period concerned me."

"As early as high school, I consulted a gynecologist about not having my period, but the message was, 'Don't worry, you're just late.' "

A girl's body begins to change noticeably even before she has her first period. She experiences a growth spurt, her breasts develop, her pubic and underarm hair grows, and her body becomes rounder in places where fat is deposited. Her first period usually comes after some or all of these changes, but it may not become regular or ovulatory for two years or longer.

In the United States and western Europe, the typical age of menarche (onset of menstruation) is now twelve and a half, which is somewhat sooner than it was twenty years ago. Experts speculate that this drop in menarche age may be due to improved living conditions, better nutrition, or better healthcare. It may be that children are reaching their full size sooner, achieving a greater weight for their height, or becoming fit and capable of childbearing at a younger age.

In this era of relatively young menarche, it's natural for a girl to become concerned when her first period is delayed. A number of factors may come into play in causing a girl's first period to be "late." Extreme thinness, serious illness, poor nutritional practices, and even the mother's age at menarche may be involved. Some physically active girls who maintain heavy training throughout adolescence may not get their first period until they are in their late teens or even early twenties. This absence of menarche may also be accompanied by a lack of secondary sex characteristics, such as the development of breasts and body hair.

Researchers have been studying the link between heavy physical activity and delayed menarche for several years. One of the original theories on delayed menarche in physically active girls was developed by Dr. Rose Frisch at the Harvard Center for Population Studies. Dr. Frisch's hypothesis was that a girl had to reach a certain weight for her particular height before her periods would begin. Dr. Frisch and her colleagues also took body composition into account. They knew that estrogen—a key hormone in the menstruation cycle—is activated and stored in fatty tissues. They therefore theorized that specific amounts of body fat were necessary for menarche to occur, and predicted that periods would begin when a girl reached a body composition of about 17 percent fat.

While it had been generally accepted that a certain amount of body fat was necessary for menarche to occur, researchers now doubt that there is a particular body fat percentage or exact weight/height ratio at which menstrual cycles begin. Eugenie C. Scott of the Department of Anthropology at the University of Kentucky in Lexington, and Francis E. Johnston of the Department of Anthropology at the University of Pennsylvania in Philadelphia, find several problems with the theory. First, measurement of body fat is an inexact science, and researchers are compelled to use estimates in determining "fat" and "lean" body weights. Second, exceptions to this theory have been established, both above and below the critical threshold. Finally, other factors, such as diet or exercise patterns, have been found to contribute to menstrual patterns and menarche which are equally acceptable in explaining the delay of menses. Labeling such an arbitrary point might be a source of worry to many girls. A more sensible approach might be to look at all the various factors that could impact menarche. Is a girl training intensely in her sport? Is she eating well? Is she maintaining or gaining weight as she grows? What about levels of stress and general health? All these factors may play a part in delaying her menarche.

Up to a certain point, we advise girls and their parents to let nature take its course, and accept a certain amount of lateness as natural for that girl. However, if a girl has not exhibited any secondary sex characteristics by about age fourteen, or has not experienced any menstrual cycles by age sixteen, she might want to consult with her healthcare provider. According to a few recent studies, very prolonged delays in menarche may result in thinning of the bones, which may ultimately put the girl at a greater risk of osteoporosis.

To understand how bones become "thin," it helps to know something about the way our bones grow. Bones are constantly undergoing a process of buildup and breakdown (resorption). Estrogen, the hormone that increases with menarche, is one of the factors that slows bone resorption so bones can have a chance to become thicker, stronger, and thus less resistant to fractures. The teens and twenties are prime times for a woman to build her skeleton to its peak. To help bolster this bone-building process, a girl with delayed periods may want to increase her dietary calcium. She should also account for the fact that some foods, like caffeine present in soft drinks, chocolate, tea, and coffee, can actually increase calcium excretion in urine (see page 172). One way to counteract this effect is to eat a balanced diet with plenty of calcium-rich foods.

LUTEAL PHASE DEFECT AND ANOVULATION

> "When my running mileage was higher, my periods were much lighter and occurred less often. I suspect that I was not ovulating during those times, but never took my temperature to confirm it."

> "When I first started running my periods were less regular, but eventually they became regular again."

If you have even been intensely active for a period of time (when training for a big event, for instance), you might have noticed a progression of changes from regular menstrual functioning to menstrual irregularity. At first, perhaps you had less intense premenstrual symptoms or a light flow. If you experienced the next steps in the progression—luteal phase defeat and anovulation—chances are you may not have noticed them.

Luteal phase defect shortens the length of time between ovulation and the onset of bleeding, a phase that would normally take fourteen days. In the case of *anovulation*, the cycle progresses normally, but no egg is released. The most serious consequences of these menstrual irregularities

r the woman who is trying to become pregnant. Certainly if a
oes not ovulate month after month, she will not become preg-
oman experiencing shortened luteal phases may also experience
fficulties. There is also some concern about possible health risks
with these conditions, because both involve some lowering of
vels. In prolonged instances of anovulation or luteal phase de-
may be some loss of bone mass. Keep in mind, however, that
els may be only slightly lowered by these conditions, and that
s also may be contributing to lower bone density.

omen don't realize they have luteal phase defect or anovula-
the overall length or nature of their cycle doesn't change
. To actually measure the length of your luteal phase, you
need to know if and when you ovulate. Taking your basal body temperature each morning for several months can help you pinpoint ovulation.
It is important to take temperature readings before getting out of bed in
the morning—before activity causes your body temperature to rise.
Charting these temperatures on paper will allow you to see a visual trend
over the month. Generally your temperature will be under 98° F during
the first part of your cycle, or follicular phase. Just before ovulation, your
temperature will dip, and then it will rise over the next day or two.
Throughout the second part, or luteal phase, your temperature will be
above 98° F.

In addition to charting, you might find it helpful to note physical
changes such as pain and tenderness in the pelvic area, called "mittel-
schmerz," that occur during the middle of your cycle. Cervical mucus will become thinner, more copious, and clear just before and during
ovulation. Usually, if you have not ovulated, you will also not have
premenstrual symptoms such as breast tenderness, mood changes, or
bloating.

Laura took her basal body temperatures for four months to determine
if she was ovulating. She was trying to become pregnant, and had heard
that as a long-distance runner she might have problems conceiving. Laura
found that the cyclic changes in her cervical mucus coincided with her
temperature charts, indicating that she was ovulating each month. For
the first twelve days of her cycle, the discharge was whitish and somewhat
thick. As ovulation approached and before her temperature rose, it be-

came thinner and clear for several days. Some months, Laura also had a light pain in her lower abdomen indicating that she had ovulated. Laura only needed to use the chart for four months; since then, she's been able to tell if she's ovulating by paying attention to the physical signs.

On the following page is a chart you can use for keeping basal body temperatures. Day one of the chart should correspond to the first day of your menstrual flow. The numbers along the left side represent tenths of a degree in temperature. To record each day's temperature, place a dot at the point where the lines for the temperature and the day intersect. Calendar dates may be placed along the top of the chart for ease of recording.

A single month of charting is not enough to give you an accurate picture of your normal menstrual cycle. If you are trying to detect anovulation or shortened luteal phase, you'll want to keep records for several months. If you do find a pattern of irregularity, the next question is, "How long should I wait before I consult a doctor?"

Researchers and physicians are divided as to the nature of menstrual disorders. Many look at menstrual irregularities in a disease framework and urge women to seek immediate medical attention. Others view menstrual changes and irregularities as the body's adaptive response to high levels of physical stress in the form of athletic training (see discussion on page 94). The natural change in hormonal levels brought on by intense workouts can alter the balance necessary to maintain regular menstrual cycles. Some researchers, including Dr. Jerilynn Prior from the University of British Columbia, believe that these changes may be the way the body conserves energy for intense physical effort.

While menstrual irregularity is a natural response, it may not feel comfortable to you, especially if it interferes with your plans to get pregnant. If obvious menstrual changes and irregularities have been continuing for many months, we feel it is wise to consult your healthcare provider. A few months of charted records will be useful in the consultations, especially if you are trying to become pregnant. Most physicians will begin fertility workups after a couple has been trying unsuccessfully to become pregnant for one year. Having charts may determine the possible cause of infertility, saving time and money by avoiding the need for other diagnostic testing.

BASAL BODY TEMPERATURE CHART

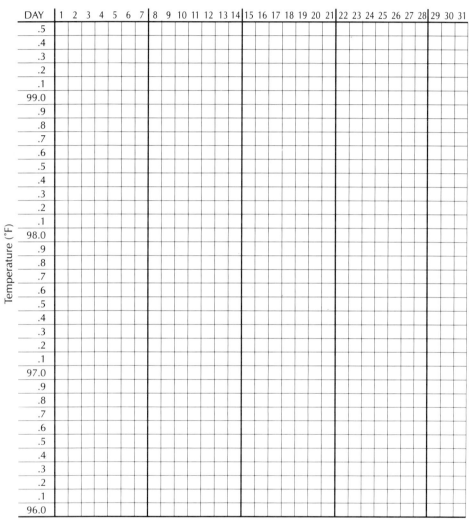

What can you expect in terms of treatment? Many researchers and physicians believe that menstrual irregularities are reversible through changes in training and lifestyle. A first step might be to decrease training time, intensity, or training patterns. A day or two off from training each week may be enough to regulate an irregular cycle. It may also be that your specific activity is affecting your cycle more than other activities would. If you are a runner, for instance, your doctor may ask you to substitute swimming or cycling for a while to see if that affects your menstrual pattern. He or she may also ask you to gain a moderate amount of weight through a sensible, nutritious diet. Before you begin any treatment plan, be sure to ask questions and become aware of all your options so you can make the best decision concerning your health.

ATHLETIC AMENORRHEA

"I feel healthy, but it worries me that I am not having a period."

"I just wanted to know why I wasn't getting my periods and if it was something to be concerned about."

"When I began running regularly I was on birth control pills and had regular periods. Since going off the pill I have only had a couple of light periods in four and a half years."

"I was worried at first about not getting my period."

Perhaps the most disconcerting menstrual change for the physically active woman is that of athletic amenorrhea, or the absence of menstrual periods. Researchers and physicians still cannot say exactly how many missed periods constitute amenorrhea. Some feel that three missed periods is considered amenorrhea, whereas others feel that true amenorrhea is a total loss of menstrual periods for at least six months, or even a year.

The concept of athletic amenorrhea, or the absence of menstrual periods associated with physical activity, moved into the spotlight during the fitness boom of the late 1970s. As more women became physically active, interest and research in this area accelerated. Reports of the possible connection between loss of periods and exercise alarmed many women who were already exercising and deterred others from starting a physical activity program.

A decade later, researchers are still struggling to pinpoint the actual cause of athletic amenorrhea. At first, researchers suspected that thinness combined with intense activity may have been primarily responsible. Today, researchers are looking at the role of the hypothalamus, an organ at the base of the brain that controls the glandular systems in the body. Hypothalamic rhythm may be altered by intense physical training, perhaps as a way for the body to conserve energy. It may be that these glandular changes cause the body to produce fewer ovary-stimulating hormones; in turn, the ovaries produce less estrogen. Lower estrogen could be one of the many factors that causes amenorrhea or oligomenorrhea (infrequent periods). Body fat, nutrition, and even stress can also exert an influence on menstrual cycles, making it difficult for us to say for sure which factor is responsible for irregularities.

BODY FAT AND BODY WEIGHT

"I quit menstruating right after a combination of weight loss and also starting endurance activity on a regular basis."

"It seems my cycle stops under stress—a weight gain or loss of more than five pounds, pressure from work, or travel."

As a result of early research, physicians and athletes are sometimes quick to blame low body weight and low body fat for the loss of periods. New research has upset this notion, however, by suggesting that other factors may be just as important. In a 1985 study at the University of Colorado, Charlotte Sanborn, Bruce Albrecht, and Wiltz Wagner, Jr., compared women who had athletic amenorrhea to women who were menstruating regularly. The two groups were similar in age, height, weight, percent body fat, and training. With all these similarities, why is it that some of these women lost their periods, whereas others did not?

Some researchers speculate that the distribution of body fat may have a greater influence on reproductive function than simply the amount of body fat. Kelly Brownell and his colleagues at the University of Pennsylvania School of Medicine advance the theory that both animals and humans have certain fat deposits that are necessary to provide energy for both pregnancy and lactation. In humans, this lactational fat is found on the hips, thighs, and buttocks. When these fat stores are depleted, as in high levels of physical training, menstrual dysfunction may result.

NUTRITION

"I continued running, but added a little fat to my diet. My periods resumed within six months."

"I have been a strict vegetarian for over nine years now, eating no red meat or fish. My periods are either irregular or nonexistent. I have seen a gynecologist about this matter earlier in the year and he attributed my 'disorder' to a high level of exercise."

At Melpomene, we were interested in finding out what part nutrition played in the maintenance of menstrual periods. We asked groups of amenorrheic and regularly menstruating athletes to keep track of their diets as well as their physical activity patterns. We found that the amenorrheic athletes ate an average of 450 calories less per day than regularly menstruating athletes. The interesting thing was that these women seemed to be able to maintain their weight on this lowered intake.

We suspect that this weight maintenance may be due to the phenomenon of food efficiency. Food efficiency is an adaptive process whereby the body adjusts to lower caloric intakes by making the most of the calories it is given. People with enhanced food efficiency can function and maintain their current weight even though they seem to be eating too little. For example, Andrea weighs 120 pounds, rows two hours each day, and consumes 1,500 calories daily. Barbara also weighs 120 pounds, rows two hours each day, but consumes only 800 calories daily. Both Andrea and Barbara are maintaining their current weight of 120 pounds. Barbara is more food efficient, however, because she is able to maintain her weight and her high level of physical activity on far fewer calories than Andrea.

Brownell speculates that food efficiency may be an adaptive trait in human beings, designed to carry a person through a biologically taxing time (e.g., famine). He and his colleagues state: "For theoretical reasons, we would expect food efficiency to be enhanced in athletes with low or fluctuating weights. These patterns may be perceived as a threat to energy stores, thus increased efficiency could be the defense. The effect should be most pronounced in athletes who are furthest below their non-training weight. The effect may be stronger in females than males because their reproductive function is more readily threatened by changes in energy stores." When a cave woman had to survive a winter of low food rations, for example, it would be beneficial for her metabolism to slow down so that she could survive on less food. Perhaps the body interprets intense exercise as another kind of environmental stress. It makes good biological sense not to bring a child into the world when food shortages are low and energy outputs are high; pregnancy and lactation simply take too much energy. In this light, the disruption of periods can also be seen as an adaptive/protective response to stress.

On the average, the women in our amenorrhea study who were the most food efficient were also amenorrheic. Other studies on athletes and nutrition have concurred with our findings, pointing to the need for pregnant women to consume an adequate number of calories if they want to maintain general good health while meeting the increased energy needs of physical training.

Vegetarianism has also been studied for its possible link to athletic amenorrhea. Many researchers, including Susan M. Brooks et al., at the University of Colorado; Patricia A. Deuster et al., at the University of Maryland; and Karl M. Pirke et al., in a West German study, have found a high number of vegetarians among the amenorrheic women whom they study. In our study, 85 percent of the amenorrheic women said they did not eat red meat; only 25 percent of the regularly menstruating women made the same statement. Some researchers feel that vegetarianism may affect the hormones that influence the menstrual cycle in two ways. First, these women may not be getting enough dietary fat, which is important for estrogen production and storage. Second, it is possible that vegetarian women eat more fiber than nonvegetarian women, and are more likely to excrete estrogen in their feces.

Another interesting finding from the Melpomene study was that the amenorrheic women were eating three to four times more vitamin A than the regularly menstruating women were eating. Beta carotene, which is a form of vitamin A found in plants and vegetables, is stored in fat cells and in the corpus luteum (in the ovaries). Researchers hypothesize that the excessive levels of beta carotene in the fat cells of very lean women may interfere with estrogen production. It is also possible that high levels of deposited beta carotene in the ovaries of these women may affect their menstrual cycles.

PHYSICAL ACTIVITY

"When I injured my knee and had to stop running for a while, menstruation returned."

"I have cut back a little on the number of miles I run each week."

It may not be how long or how intensely you work out that causes a change in your menstrual cycle. The real disruption seems to occur when you change your level of activity abruptly. A woman who goes from doing nothing to running several miles a day, for instance, may be more likely to develop menstrual problems than the woman who slowly works up to that level of activity.

The sport you choose to participate in may also affect your menstrual patterns. Studies have shown that there is a higher incidence of amenorrhea in "thin-person" sports than in sports where weight does not matter. Menstrual problems are found to be more common, for instance, in women who participate in distance running, ballet, and gymnastics. In contrast, swimmers have a fairly low incidence of amenorrhea or menstrual changes, which is due partly to the higher levels of body fat that swimmers maintain for regulating body temperature in the water.

Very high levels of training have also been found to be a factor in athletic amenorrhea, especially when the training program is just starting. Over time, the body may adapt to the high levels of activity, but initially the high energy expenditure and possible lowering of body weight/fat may be enough to disrupt periods.

THE EFFECTS OF LONG-TERM ATHLETIC AMENORRHEA

> "What concerns me is prolonged amenorrhea. I am married and may someday be interested in having children and am curious if this will present problems."

Two questions most women ask about their own amenorrhea are "Is it harmful to me?" and "Will it affect my fertility?" For many years, scientists and physicians were divided as to the long-term effects of athletic amenorrhea. Then in the early 1980s, researchers found that athletes who did not have menstrual periods seemed to be losing mineral content in their bones, which may put them at risk for osteoporosis. The phenomenon of bone tissue loss is normal and occurs in each of us, but it is usually offset by bone buildup—a balance that keeps our bones strong. One of the key ingredients in this balance is estrogen, the hormone that controls the rate of bone loss through resorption. Without estrogen to slow bone loss, the balance was thrown out of whack, and the athletes studied began seeing a net loss in bone density, especially in their spine. This was somewhat surprising considering that muscle activity through exercise is known to actually increase total bone mass. Evidently, exercise was not enough to offset the bone loss caused by the lowered estrogen.

Bone loss is also apparent in menopausal women, who may lose up to 2 percent of their bone mass per year for the first four to five years after menopause. The rate of bone loss continues in the later postmenopausal years, but usually at a slower rate. The loss of estrogen is also the probable cause of bone loss in premenopausal women who have had their ovaries removed.

But there is good news. Dr. Barbara Drinkwater of the Pacific Medical Center in Seattle, Washington, one of the early researchers to explore the link between bone loss and amenorrhea, conducted a study of amenorrheic women who had resumed their menstrual cycles. She found that their bone density increased after their cycles began again. This finding is especially important for younger women athletes, who are able to continue to build bone density in their twenties and early thirties. The older amenorrheic athlete may want to seek medical intervention, however, since she is not as readily able to rebuild lost bone density after about age thirty-five.

A second concern for the amenorrheic athlete is fertility. Many women who have stopped having periods are worried that they won't be able to get pregnant. While it's true that you can't get pregnant if you are not ovulating, it's also true the amenorrhea can reverse itself at any time. You may skip your period for three months and then suddenly ovulate and menstruate in the fourth month.

Once a woman starts ovulating and menstruating again, the fact that she was once amenorrheic does not seem to have any effect on her fertility. As long as she starts ovulating at midcycle, she is capable of conceiving children. Amenorrhea, like an oral contraceptive, merely causes a time-out in reproductive functioning. Once reversed, regular reproductive functioning should resume. (Because you can't predict when ovulation might resume again, it's not a good idea to use amenorrhea as a form of birth control!)

If you are having regular periods after having been amenorrheic, and you are still unable to get pregnant, it may be that you are not ovulating midcycle. Outwardly, your cycle can seem completely normal, but if you don't release an egg, you won't be able to get pregnant. It is also common to experience infrequent periods in the transition from amenorrhea to regular cycles. Charting basal body temperatures will help you to determine if you are ovulating. Again, this procedure is a helpful tool when consulting your physician about fertility problems.

TREATMENT FOR ATHLETIC AMENORRHEA

"I had one period last year, and it was brought on by the use of prescribed drugs."

"I am willing to slow down the running; so far I've been replacing it with more swimming."

"I have not had a period in four years and have cut back on my jogging. My doctor thinks estrogen/progesterone will help. I don't really care to take these hormones. Help!"

"My concern now is to regain a normal menstrual cycle so I can become pregnant. I have stopped running entirely for almost a year now. I have also increased my weight from a low of 100 pounds three years ago to 112 pounds present."

"I would like to become pregnant. I would also like not to have to give up those forty or fifty miles per week running."

"I am currently being seen by an ob/gyn who put me on birth control pills about six months ago. They seem to be working well. I'm having regular periods after six and a half years of nothing!"

Many women who develop athletic amenorrhea are not sure what to do. Some feel it is imperative to see their physician as soon as they miss a period, and others are willing to wait several months or even a year before consulting a doctor. This timetable is a matter of personal choice. However, to rule out other causes of amenorrhea, including pregnancy or pituitary malfunctions, we feel it is important to check with your physician after one missed period if you suspect pregnancy. Otherwise, most physicians feel that you should consult your doctor after three missed periods.

When it comes to treating athletic amenorrhea, the experts fall into two camps. Some feel that it is important to treat amenorrhea immediately to avoid possible problems with bone demineralization or fertility. Others have a wait-and-see attitude. They believe that athletic amenorrhea is the body's way of adapting to the extra stresses of physical training, lower caloric consumption, or a change in body composition. They contend that in most cases, amenorrhea will reverse itself without intervention.

When consulting your physician about amenorrhea, he or she should perform the following procedures to determine the cause before beginning any sort of treatment plan:

1. Collect or update your health information and history, which should include a history of dieting or weight loss, amount and intensity of exercise, a nutritional assessment, and any past health and reproductive problems. Psychological factors such as stress should also be considered, as well as the possibility of anorexia nervosa or other eating disorders.

2. Perform a pelvic exam to observe any reproductive abnormalities or possible pregnancy.

3. If everything appears normal and you are not pregnant, he or she should order some laboratory studies that will determine your levels of hormones such as plasma prolactin. Prolactin, which is important for lactation, has been found to increase in some highly trained athletic women, and researchers believe the increase may be associated with athletic amenorrhea. Your doctor should also know about any medications you are taking, since certain medications can elevate prolactin levels. Thyroid levels should also be measured to rule out hypothyroidism (underactive thyroid), and levels of FSH and LH should be checked to determine if you are having premature ovarian failure. If prolactin is elevated, then a computerized tomography (CT) scan may be necessary to see if a pituitary tumor exists.

4. Finally, if you've been amenorrheic for a long time, he or she might want to evaluate your bone density before developing a treatment plan.

After all these tests, you and your physician may choose to do nothing while waiting to see if your periods resume naturally. Your doctor might also recommend that you trim back your training schedule, do a different activity once or twice a week (such as tennis or swimming instead of running), or eliminate speed training for a few months. Your physician may also suggest that you gain some weight. A regimen of decreased training and weight gain is not guaranteed to produce immediate results. It may take several months before your period returns, or you may discover that this change in activity level or weight gain does not improve your ability to conceive.

Another treatment for athletic amenorrhea is hormonal replacement therapy. Estrogen and/or progesterone, possibly in the form of birth control pills, may be prescribed to treat amenorrhea and to prevent bone loss. If side effects or health risks do not make this option sensible, the following regimes may be suggested by your healthcare professional. In most cases, you will take 5 to 10 mg/day of medroxyprogesterone (Amen,

Provera) for ten days each cycle and/or .625 mg/day of conjugated estrogens (Premarin) for days one through twenty-five of a cycle to prevent bone demineralization. If you have withdrawal bleeding after taking these hormones, you'll know that your outflow tract (uterus and vagina) is normal. Clomiphene citrate (Clomid) in the amount of 25 to 50 mg/day for five days beginning early in the menstrual cycle will induce ovulation and eventually menstruation. Estrogen may also be given one to two months before clomiphene citrate to help prime the uterine lining. If clomiphene citrate is not effective, other hormones, such as human chorionic gonadotropin, may be used.

Again, treatment options are a choice to be made by you and your healthcare provider. Be sure your physician is willing to answer your questions, listen to your concerns, and present and discuss all the options *before* you begin treatment. The success of a treatment depends on your makeup and health history; what works wonders for a friend of yours may not be appropriate for you. It's especially important to think carefully about hormonal replacement treatments. If you do choose to work with hormones, both you and your physician should pay close attention to any changes or side effects that may occur.

PREMENSTRUAL SYNDROME (PMS)

"Usually, the day before I get my period I have extreme highs and lows in my mood."

"I get irritable and emotional two to three days before I begin menstruating."

"Two weeks before the onset of my period, I have severe melancholy and lethargy. Getting my period is a relief."

"I am inclined to binge on chocolate prior to my flow if I'm not paying attention."

"I'm much more active in the summer and I notice significantly fewer mood swings and less physical pain around menstruation."

Many women go through cyclical changes a few days before their period. Their moods may fluctuate, their breasts may be sore, or perhaps they feel bloated with a few extra pounds of "water weight." For 10 percent of all menstruating women, these physical and psychological changes can be severe enough to disrupt their lives. Premenstrual syndrome, or PMS, is experienced by 40 percent of all women who menstruate. Despite its prevalence, PMS is still the subject of much controversy in the medical community. Scientists and physicians can't seem to agree on an exact definition, or even whether PMS is a discreet syndrome. One problem is that the symptoms are so wide-ranging that it's difficult to tie them to a single syndrome. Finally, although some treatments work for some symptoms (e.g., nutritional therapies can ease depression), there is no treatment for PMS that is consistently effective for all symptoms.

No one really knows what causes PMS. Most researchers believe that hormonal change or imbalance is the culprit. One popular theory is that PMS is linked to an imbalance in the ratio of progesterone to estrogen. It is also possible that PMS is actually more than one syndrome, with different causes for each symptom or group of symptoms. This theory would explain why no single treatment is effective for all symptoms or all women.

In general, PMS occurs every month and is cyclical in nature. Symptoms appear during the luteal phase (last half) of the cycle and should lessen once the menstrual period begins. Then at least one symptom-free week should occur. Finally, PMS should not be confused with dysmenorrhea, which is characterized by pain and cramping during menstrual periods.

SYMPTOMS

PMS encompasses a wide range of symptoms, both physical and psychological. Bloating is the most common physical symptom, but breast tenderness, swelling, pelvic pain, headache, and bowel changes are also common. Irritability and aggressiveness are some of the most common psychological symptoms of PMS. Others include depression, anxiety, lack of concentration, appetite changes, tension, change in sex drive, and insomnia.

Below is a scheme for categorizing PMS symptoms as proposed by endocrinologist Dr. Guy Abraham. The initials PMT (premenstrual tension) are followed by *A* for anxiety, *C* for carbohydrate craving and intolerance, *H* for hyperhydration or water retention, and *D* for depression.

PMTA (ANXIETY) AFFECTS 80 PERCENT OF PMS SUFFERERS

Nervous tension
Mood swings
Irritability
Anger
Anxiety
Depression

PMTC (CARBOHYDRATE CRAVING AND INTOLERANCE) AFFECTS 60 PERCENT OF PMS SUFFERERS

Headache
Sweet cravings
Alcohol cravings
Increased appetite
Heart pounding
Fatigue
Dizziness
Faintness

PMTH (HYPERHYDRATION OR WATER RETENTION) AFFECTS 40 PERCENT OF PMS SUFFERERS

Weight gain
Swelling of extremities
Breast tenderness
Abdominal bloating

PMTD (DEPRESSION) AFFECTS 20 PERCENT OF PMS SUFFERERS

Severe depression
Withdrawal
Confusion
Crying easily
Insomnia
Forgetfulness
Suicidal thoughts

A good way to determine if you suffer from PMS is to chart your symptoms. Keeping a menstrual calendar or chart like the one on page 107 can help you determine which symptoms are cyclic, when they occur, and whether they are in fact premenstrual. A chart should include (1) the days you menstruate, (2) the days that symptoms occur, (3) the symptom, and (4) the severity of the symptom. Recording your basal body temperature each day (see page 93) can be especially helpful in determining when you ovulate and when you are premenstrual. You might also find it useful to keep track of your physical activity level and how you feel on certain days of your cycle in relation to your exercise program.

After three or four months of charting, you may see patterns emerge that will help you identify your problem and target your treatment. Try grouping the symptoms that you see cropping up into either physical or psychological categories (e.g., bloating and breast tenderness would be physical symptoms, while anxiety, depression, and frequent crying would be psychological). If symptoms are disabling or severe enough to be interfering with your life, and you do seek treatment, this grouping will help your physician prescribe the most effective treatment for you.

TREATMENT OF PMS

While many of the women affected by PMS do not need treatment, there are some who are debilitated by symptoms each month. For these women, treatment may significantly improve the quality of their lives. Drug therapies for PMS include hormonal interventions (progesterone is the most

PREMENSTRUAL SYMPTOMS CHART

Grading of Symptoms

0 NONE
1 MILD: present but does not interfere with activities
2 MODERATE: present and interferes with activities but not disabling
3 SEVERE: disabling, unable to function

DATE	1	2	3	4	5	6	7	8	9	10	11	12	13	14	15	16	17	18	19	20	21	22	23	24	25	26	27	28	29	30	31
Basal weight																															
Basal body tempeature																															
Menstruation																															
Day of cycle																															
Nervous tension																															
Mood swings																															
Irritabliity																															
Anxiety																															
Headache																															
Cravings																															
Increased appetite																															
Nausea																															
Depression																															
Forgetfulness																															
Crying																															
Confusion																															
Clumsiness																															
Insomnia																															
Weight gain																															
Swelling																															
Breast tenderness																															
Bloating																															
Cramps																															
Backache																															
General aches & pains																															
Diarrhea																															
Constipation																															
Skin changes																															
Allergies																															
Infections																															
Other symptoms:																															
Treatments:																															
Physical activity:																															

Source. Adapted from the Women's Health Clinic, Winnepeg, Manatoba Canada.

107

widely used) and diuretics. Nonhormonal treatments range from diet or vitamin therapy to stress reduction exercises and massage.

Most experts agree that physical activity can have some value in relieving PMS symptoms. Dr. Jerilyn Prior at the University of British Columbia found that stress and anxiety were decreased in groups of women who had begun exercise, or who had increased training levels. The women in the study who were not training did not experience these improvements.

Aerobic activity, in which the heart rate is increased, seems to alleviate PMS symptoms better than nonaerobic activity. The increase in circulation associated with aerobic exercise can decrease bloating and fluid buildup, while the beta-endorphins responsible for "runner's high" can help lighten or calm your mood. Physical activity also relieves muscular tension, helps lessen joint pain, and changes abnormal patterns often associated with PMS. Finally, regular exercise increases the effectiveness of insulin, which helps the body convert starches and sugars into energy. This fast and efficient digestion helps stabilize blood sugar levels and helps decrease food cravings during the premenstrual stage.

CONTRACEPTION AND PHYSICALLY ACTIVE WOMEN

"I am concerned about putting on weight if I go on the pill. I am also worried about the emotional side effects."

"I have found that barrier methods of contraception have had the least impact on my physical activities."

"I have been using oral contraceptives for over ten years and have not experienced any menstrual irregularities as a result of running. Will either one make it any easier or more difficult for me to conceive, if and when I choose to do so?"

Most physically active women are health-conscious and committed to making decisions that enhance their health and well-being. Women faced with contraceptive choices are often undecided as to which method is best for them. Most women are looking for a safe, effective method of contraception that poses no health risks and will not jeopardize future fertility. Women who are active may be concerned with how side effects will affect their athletic endeavors, or how birth control devices will stand up to the rigors of intense activity.

More and more physically active women are choosing barrier methods of contraception, such as the diaphragm, cervical cap, condoms, or contraceptive foam or jelly. Barrier methods give the women more control over contraception with minimal side effects. Also, barrier methods do not interfere with the body's hormonal system, nor do they interfere with physical activity for the most part. Diaphragms, however, must be left in for six hours after intercourse and may therefore need to be left in during exercise. If discomfort results from wearing a diaphragm during physical activity, a smaller-size diaphragm may be necessary. Other negative aspects of barrier methods include their inconvenience; some women and their partners also complain about the lack of spontaneity associated with this kind of contraception.

Athletes tend to avoid using the intrauterine device (IUD) as a method of contraception. Although the IUD does not alter hormonal balance, the possible side effects deter most physically active women. Complications associated with the IUD are heavier periods, dysmenorrhea, and risk of pelvic inflammatory disease, which may cause infertility.

The rhythm method of contraception requires charting of basal body temperature and changes in cervical mucus in order to find out fertile times. Athletes who experience menstrual irregularities such as anovulatory cycles and shortened luteal phase will find that the rhythm method is unreliable. In the same way, amenorrhea is not an effective form of birth control. As we mentioned before, you never know when ovulation will occur.

Oral contraceptives or birth control pills present the greatest dilemma for women, because there are both benefits and risks associated with their use. They are convenient, produce regular menstrual cycles, and often decrease dysmenorrhea. Also, oral contraceptives provide enough estrogen to prevent bone loss in those women who are at risk. Despite its advantages, the pill does have its share of negative side effects. In general, there is a four times greater risk of cardiovascular problems, deep vein thrombosis (blood clots), or stroke in women who take birth control pills than in non-pill users. Five out of every 100,000 women who use the pill die from these complications each year. The chance for problems increases with women who smoke, who are over age thirty-five, and for those who have been on the pill for many years. For women under thirty-five years who do not smoke, the mortality rate falls to 0.7 per 100,000 women per year. For athletic women, the risks may be even lower due to lower body weight, lower body fat, and the fact that athletic women are aerobically conditioned—all factors that lower the risk of cardiovascular disease. Also, most physically active women do not smoke.

Active women often want to know if birth control pills will affect their athletic performance. While there is little research in this area, preliminary findings indicate that oral contraceptives may lead to a decrease in athletic performance. One study found that maximal oxygen uptake (one measure of fitness) was lowered during bicycle exercise in women who were taking oral contraceptives compared to women who were not taking the pills. Another study found that when exercising, women who were on oral contraceptives reached the point of exhaustion faster than those who were not taking the pill. Possible weight gain due to water retention is another reason some athletes steer away from the pill. New, lower-dose oral contraceptives are gaining popularity, however, in part because they produce less fluid retention and weight gain than the earlier birth control pills did.

Another concern for women contemplating the pill is the possibility of increasing their risk of cancer. When oral contraceptives were first introduced, research showed no increase in breast cancer in the short-term, but these studies were unable to predict the long-term effects of taking the pill. Current research is still showing no increase in breast cancer in the general population of women on oral contraceptives, but certain subgroups of women are considered at higher risk. These subgroups include women with a personal or family history of breast cancer and women with a previous history of benign breast disease. The consensus of opinion from a Centers for Disease Control (CDC) study and also from the Food and Drug Administration (FDA) is that oral contraceptives have not been clearly implicated as an independent risk factor for breast cancer. However results from a 1989 study in Sweden showed an increase in the risk of breast cancer among women who were receiving hormone replacement therapy, especially among those who were taking progesterone. This study, conducted by Leif Bergkvist and his colleagues at the University Hospital in Uppsala, Sweden, is neither conclusive, nor does it study women who are actually taking oral contraceptives. But this study is important because it raises questions, and points to a need for further study of the relationship between hormones and breast cancer. Endometrial (uterine lining) cancer seems to be even less of a threat; in fact, some experts suspect that the balance between estrogen and progesterone in the pills may actually decrease the risk of endometrial cancer. The important thing to remember about these reports, however, is that they are speculative; the true long-term effects of oral contraceptives will not be known until the product has been in use for quite a long period of time.

The chart below summarizes the various contraceptive methods, as well as some of their advantages, disadvantages, and considerations for physical activity:

Method	Pregnancy Rate* (percent)	Restrictions on Physical Activity
Abstinence	0	None.
Coitus interruptus	20–25	May lead to pregnancy.
Rhythm method	5–30	None. Increased awareness of body.
Symptothermal method (Similar to rhythm method. Involves taking basal body temperature)	10–40	None. Increased awareness of body.
Condom	2–10	None.
Diaphragm	2–10	Few. Should stay in place while exercising. May be uncomfortable exercising with diaphragm in place.
Sponge	10–20	Few. Should stay in place during physical activity.
Foams/Jellies	15–20	Can be messy.
Cervical cap (Similar to diaphragm)	5–13	Few. Should stay in place during physical activity.
Intrauterine device (IUD)	5	Pain, bleeding, and complications may interfere with physical activity.

Method	Pregnancy Rate* (percent)	Restrictions on Physical Activity
Combination birth control pills	1–2	Possible water-weight gain and other bodily changes. May affect physical performance.
Progestin-only birth control pills	1–3	Irregular menstruation can be very inconvenient for physically active women. Bodily changes may affect performance.

Source: A compilation of information from the Boston Women's Health Book Collective, Dr. Jerilyn Prior, and a membership survey conducted by the Melpomene Staff.
*Failure rate per 100 women per year. Low number represents theoretical failure rate. High number represents actual failure rate of women who use the method correctly and consistently.

In choosing a method of contraception, you will also want to consider the effectiveness of the method you will use. Clearly, some forms of contraception are more effective than others. For example, the actual effectiveness rate of barrier methods ranges from 10 percent to 15 percent failure rate per 100 women per year of use compared to a failure rate of 2 percent to 4 percent for birth control pills.

Whatever contraceptive method you decide on, we recommend that you consider not only its effectiveness but also its impact on your health, lifestyle, and future fertility. In the final analysis, you are the best judge of what feels right for you, and therefore only you can make decisions about your health.

In this chapter, we've looked at the many changes, both major and minor, that can alter your menstrual cycle. Physical activity can on the one hand help improve your health, but on the other hand, it may at some point affect your menstrual patterns. A number of other lifestyle factors such as diet and stress may also have an effect on your cycle. Keep in mind that while your cycle variations may not be average or what is considered "normal," these variations are not necessarily unhealthy, and may in fact be quite common among other women who are enjoying a physically active lifestyle.

F O U R

PREGNANCY AND FITNESS

Say you've recently discovered the joys of exercise (or maybe you've always been a believer), and suddenly, you're asked to stop. You're told to put your feet up for nine months and be careful. But you know you're not sick, and you haven't had an injury! Yet this news greets many pregnant women.

IS IT SAFE TO EXERCISE WHILE PREGNANT?

We frequently hear from women who have been told to cut back or quit exercising completely. An ultramarathoner calls to say, "I'm two months pregnant and my doctor has told me that running pounds the baby, so I stopped running. But I'm bored! Can't I run just a little?" If you are pregnant, or contemplating motherhood, you'll naturally have questions about your own exercise program. Is it safe? How will it affect you? How will it affect your baby?

We are not, of course, the first generation of women who have been concerned about the effects of physical labor and activity on the outcome of our pregnancies. Women throughout the world have been active during their term. Exodus 1:19 states, "The Hebrew women are not as the Egyptian women; for they are lively, and are delivered ere the midwife come unto them."

More recent historical references are full of both admonitions and warnings about exercising during pregnancy. An 1888 treatise entitled *Wife and Mother, or, Information for Every Woman*, coauthored by physicians Pye Henry Chavasse and Sarah Hackett Stevenson, notes, "Exercise, fresh air

113

and occupation are then essentially necessary in pregnancy. If they be neglected, hard and tedious labors are likely to ensue." On the other hand, the same authors warn, "Stooping, lifting of heavy weights, and overreaching ought to be carefully avoided. Running, horseback riding, and dancing are likewise dangerous—they frequently induce a miscarriage."

Do we know more than the people of biblical times? Do we have any better advice today than we had in 1888? Today, pregnant women are still asking if they can exercise without harming their baby, and the answers they get are far from consistent. In a Melpomene study of pregnant runners and swimmers, more than 90 percent of these women said that their healthcare provider was supportive of their desire to exercise while pregnant. In a comparable group of nonexercising pregnant women, however, only 60 percent said their healthcare provider made positive comments about exercise and pregnancy. Neither group of professionals was able to fully answer questions about exercise and pregnancy, nor could they supply specific information. Only about 75 percent of the exercising pregnant women believed their providers to be knowledgeable about the issue.

Why isn't research information more readily available? One reason is that we are limited in the kind of laboratory research that we can conduct on human beings. A pregnant woman, for instance, cannot remain in a lab for nine months while we study her under controlled conditions. Naturally, the outcome of pregnancy will be based on many factors, of which exercise is only one. There are also ethical questions to consider when studying humans beings. Would it be right to knowingly cause a mother to overexert herself so that we could see what effect it has on the baby? That price would obviously be too high for anyone to pay. Instead, we look at tests made on laboratory animals, but these findings are not necessarily valid for women.

This lack of information prompted us to begin, in 1983, a descriptive study of pregnant, exercising women in a natural, rather than a laboratory, setting. We asked seventy-seven runners and twenty-seven swimmers to complete a series of questionnaires during their term. They recorded their medical histories, patterns of exercise, nutrition, discomfort, and finally, their labor and delivery experiences. We also followed a group of twenty-seven nonexercising women so we could compare their experiences during pregnancy, labor, and delivery with those of the exercising women. At two months and six months after their babies were born we checked on each woman's health and exercise patterns as well as her child's health and development.

Here are some of the things we found:

1. The women who exercised did not experience any more miscarriages, or infant or fetal deaths than the general population.
2. Twenty-two percent of the women who exercised had cesarean sections, which is comparable to the general population.
3. The women who exercised gained less weight than the women who did not exercise. On the average, runners gained 25 pounds, swimmers gained 27 pounds, and nonexercising women gained 31 pounds.
4. Labors were similar for all three groups.
5. The average weights of all the infants were in the normal range. On the average, babies born to swimmers weighed 7 pounds 2 ounces, those of runners weighed 7 pounds 9 ounces, and those of nonexercising women weighed 7 pounds 14 ounces.
6. APGAR scores, a measure of newborn well-being, were similar for all groups.
7. The main benefits of exercising during pregnancy were psychological. As one woman wrote, "Exercise gives me an alive feeling—pregnancy is a natural state; you are limited, but by no means incapable. My spirits soared as I walked and dreamed and talked to our baby. You get more oxygen and so does the baby. Inactivity causes a vicious cycle of fatigue."
8. Runners decreased both their mileage and pace as their pregnancies progressed. Their average mileage per week in the first trimester was 21.2 miles at a pace of 8.87 minutes per mile. In the third trimester their average mileage was 7.5 miles per week at a pace of 10.68 minutes per mile.
9. Forty-one of the seventy-seven runners continued to run into the third trimester. Only two swimmers stopped before the third trimester: one because of a sinus infection and the other because she was bothered by dry skin.
10. The majority of the women in the study felt exercise to be beneficial during pregnancy, even if they were not exercising on a regular basis.

What we learned from these women, and from a 1981 Melpomene study of 195 women who ran during their pregnancies, is consistent with most other studies of the natural histories of women exercising during pregnancy. For the most part, women and their babies don't seem any worse for wear as a result of their exercise. And in fact, from a psychological standpoint, it seems that the exercising women were actually better off than their nonexercising counterparts.

The only study we could find that pointed to possible problems with exercising mothers was a 1984 study conducted in Vermont. Dr. James Clapp found that women who exercised aerobically in the third trimester had lower maternal weight gains, shorter gestational lengths, and lower birth weights than women who did not exercise, or who stopped exercising before twenty-eight weeks. Although the number of women in his sample was small, some researchers were concerned because babies with lower birth weights may be subject to health and developmental problems. That was not the case in this study, however; both mothers and babies remained healthy. These findings, by the way, have not been replicated.

Of course, this case does not mean that "anything goes" during pregnancy. For instance, a 1978 survey of 208 scuba divers suggests babies born to women who continue to dive during pregnancy have a high number of birth defects. Pressure, chilling, and a combination of other factors may have dangerous implications for pregnant scuba divers. On the other hand, Japanese and Korean pearl divers work regularly during pregnancy, and yet seem to experience no problems. These ama, who dive to depths of 80 feet and remain submerged for several minutes, do not even use diving equipment! However, the official position of the Underseas Medical Society discourages women from diving during pregnancy until further studies are completed.

Given all the conflicting opinions, how can pregnant women make decisions about exercise during pregnancy? The first step is to do just what you are doing. Find out as much as you can about exercise and pregnancy. In this chapter, we will review what is known about some of the specific issues, including cardiovascular and respiratory system responses of both mother and fetus, maternal musculoskeletal effects, thermoregulatory concerns, nutritional needs, labor and delivery experiences, and postpartum considerations.

In reviewing the available data, remember that there will always be limits to what we know. We have already mentioned the technical and ethical limits to what research can be done. In addition, what happens during a pregnancy is influenced by many personal variables, such as lifestyle and genetics, that cannot be factored into "averages." Pregnancy is different for each of us, depending on who we are and what we choose to do. Thus, listening to your own body is crucial.

HEART AND LUNG CONSIDERATIONS

Of the many anatomic and functional changes that will occur in your body during pregnancy, those in your cardiovascular and respiratory systems will show up most strikingly when you begin to exercise.

Summary of Maternal Changes with Pregnancy

Parameter	Percent Increase	Percent Decrease	Unchanged
Respiratory system			
Tidal volume	30–40		
Respiratory rate			x
Resistance of tracheobronchial tree		36	
Expiratory reserve		40	
Residual volume		40	
Functional residual capacity		25	
Vital capacity			x
Respiratory minute volume	40		
Cardiovascular system			
Heart			
Rate	0–20		
Stroke volume	x		
Cardiac output	20–30		
Blood pressure			x
Peripheral blood flow	600		
Blood volume	48		
Blood constituents			
Leukocytes	70–100		
Fibrinogen	50		

Summary of Maternal Changes with Pregnancy

Parameter	Percent Increase	Percent Decrease	Unchanged
Platelets	33		
Carbon dioxide		25	
Standard bicarbonate		10	
Proteins		15	
Lipids	33		
Phospholipids	30–40		
Cholesterol	100		
Clotting factors I, VII, VIII, IX, X, XIII	x	x	
Gastrointestinal system			
Cardiac sphincter tone		x	
Acid secretion		x	
Motility		x	
Gallbladder emptying		x	
Urinary tract			
Renal plasma flow	25–50		
Glomerular filtration rate	50		
Ureter tone		x	
Ureteral motility			x
Metabolism			
Nitrogen stores	x		
General stores of			
Sodium	x		
Potassium	x		
Calcium	x		
Oxygen consumption	14		

Source: Obstetrics and Gynecology, 3rd edition, edited by D. N. Danforth, Maternal physiology (p. 282) by E. J. Quilligan and I. H. Kaiser, 1977, Philadelphia: Harper & Row. Reprinted with permission.
Note: X means function is unchanged.

Your heart and lungs must work overtime to meet the increased energy needs of pregnancy. Your baby is growing, your own tissues are increasing, and more blood is being pumped through your body as a result of an increase in heart rate. Blood volume, the total amount of blood in your body, also increases.

Contrary to what many women think, you don't lose your fitness level during pregnancy. In fact, your oxygen consumption—a measure of fitness that is also called aerobic capacity—increases throughout your term until it is 30 percent greater than the nonpregnant level. Studies indicate that you can actually increase your aerobic capacity by exercising while you are pregnant. You may feel different when you exercise, however, because you're carrying more weight now, and it takes more energy to do the same activities you did before you were pregnant. Exercise physiologists say that activities have a higher "energy cost" during pregnancy.

You may also hyperventilate or feel breathless during pregnancy, which can be a drawback when you exercise. One runner told us, "For me, the first month was the hardest because my breathing was much more strained. Once I got used to it, the running was easier." Some of this breathlessness occurs because you are more sensitive to carbon dioxide, an effect stimulated by the increased progesterone (a hormone) in your body. Also, as your uterus grows, it pushes against your diaphragm. In response, your lower ribs flare and your chest expands in an attempt to preserve lung capacity.

In many ways the female body is adapted to handle the extra energy load associated with being pregnant. What happens, then, when we add the demands of exercise to this load? Can our hearts and lungs meet this increased demand? When we exercise, our bodies deal with stress by diverting some blood flow away from the internal tissues and toward the muscles that are doing the work. Since blood is the vehicle that carries oxygen to the fetus, researchers wonder whether strenuous exercise might divert some oxygen-filled blood away from the fetus, resulting in fetal hypoxia, or lack of oxygen.

One study, conducted more than thirty years ago by Norman Morris at the University College Hospital in London, noted a decrease in the amount of blood flowing into the uterus while women were exercising. The women in this study, however, were resting on their backs, a position that is uncomfortable in late pregnancy for good reason. While on your back, the uterus can compress the vena cava—a main artery through which blood flows from the body back to the heart. This compression naturally interferes with the amount of blood available for the heart to pump back into the uterus. In this study, we don't know how much of the decreased blood flow was actually caused by exercise, and how much was blocked by the pinched artery.

Unfortunately, we do not have a safe way directly to observe blood flow to the uterus and the fetus. Mona Shangold and James Clapp have looked at how the fetus' heart rate changes as a result of the mother's exercise. They suspect that this observation may tell us, indirectly, how much blood flow, and therefore oxygen, is reaching the fetus. Recent studies at Brown University in Providence, Rhode Island, indicate that fetal heart rate drops after the mother exercises strenuously. Babies born to these women did not seem to show any signs of hypoxia, however. These studies looked only at the effects of short periods of exercise which were defined as lasting less than thirty minutes. We still do not know how repeated, prolonged episodes of high-intensity maternal exercise might influence fetal development.

Ethical considerations keep us from studying the effects of long-term, high-intensity exercise in the lab, but the body's own defenses may keep women from engaging in this kind of activity anyway. After a while, very strenuous activity becomes quite uncomfortable for pregnant women, especially later in their term. Perhaps these discomforts are a natural safety valve—your body's way of forcing you to cut back on activity. Pregnant women themselves have commented about their voluntary change in exercise habits. One runner told us, "I don't feel bad cutting back my mileage. Now I run only for pleasure—it's a different type of running."

MUSCLE AND BONE EFFECTS

No research on exercise and pregnancy has yet been done by orthopedists or physical therapists who work most directly with the musculoskeletal system. The two major concerns for physically active women in this area are back pain and a loosening of the joints associated with pregnancy.

POSTURE AND BACK PAIN

During pregnancy, your center of gravity moves forward and upward as your baby grows and your breasts enlarge. To compensate for these changes, many women slump their shoulders and arch their backs. The resulting back curvature, called lumbar lordosis, can cause fatigue and lower back pain. About 50 percent of pregnant women experience this kind of back pain. Whether or not your back will hurt seems to have nothing to do with how much weight you gain or how much your baby weighs. There does seem to be an association, however, between back pain and maternal age and number of previous pregnancies.

We do not know for sure what role exercise plays in back problems during pregnancy. We do know that abdominal muscles help support the back as well as the uterus. Therefore, developing good abdominal muscle tone going into pregnancy may be one way to lessen backache problems. In any case, the shift in your center of gravity, as well as your increasing weight, will mean a change in balance—something you will have to be vigilantly aware of as you exercise.

If you participate in sports requiring great balance and agility, you'll need to be extra alert. A physician working with downhill skiers noticed that the first sign of pregnancy in one of her clients was a rapid deterioration in skiing ability that put her at risk for injury.

Echoing trends in the general population, half of the runners, swimmers, and nonexercising women in the Melpomene study experienced back pain during pregnancy. As with other pregnancy-related aches, pains, and physical problems, the women tried to adjust their habits to decrease these discomforts. A triathlete who participated in our research developed back pain in the second trimester, reportedly due to an uncomfortable chair at work. Since her back was particularly sore in the evenings (the only time she could exercise), she would often cut back on the duration and intensity of her workout.

Another woman who ran in the Olympic Marathon trials during her second trimester experienced lower back pain. She was accustomed to running ten miles per day but said, "I had lower back problems after running from about five months on. I had to decrease my mileage to three miles or less at a time. I learned that leaning forward while I ran helped ease the pressure." It is important to let your body be your guide.

Dr. Mona Shangold, an obstetrician/gynecologist interested in sports medicine, believes that all women, including pregnant women, should be encouraged to participate in some sort of strength training program to strengthen their upper body and help avoid back problems. The originators of one maternal fitness program have tried to combine strength training with aerobic conditioning to decrease discomfort and also to prepare women for labor and delivery. Research by Douglas Hall and David Kaufmann found that women who were pregnant for the first time were less likely to undergo a cesarean section if they participated regularly in this program. Average time in labor was not affected. All the women in the exercise program reported that they enjoyed the program, no matter what their level of participation.

SOFTENING LIGAMENTS AND CARTILAGE

The hormone relaxin, which is secreted by the corpus luteum, is detectable only in pregnant women. Relaxin causes the body's connective tissues, the ligaments and cartilage, to soften and stretch so that the pelvic outlet will be able to accommodate the baby at birth. Though this softening proves to be a great help during delivery, it may subject joints to undue strain during pregnancy. It becomes easier to turn an ankle or twist a hip, for instance, because joints are able to stretch farther than they normally would, and the stabilizing ligaments are more pliable. You'll want to be particularly careful during weight-bearing activities such as walking and running.

The round ligaments that support the uterus become stretched as the fetus grows. Some women who engage in activities such as running, in which there can be movement that tugs these ligaments, experience pain. Support from a lightweight maternity girdle, or panty girdle, can reportedly offer some relief.

Unlike muscle fiber, which is elastic, connective tissue does not regain its shape once it is stretched. As you will see in the diagram, your abdominal muscles are joined in the middle by a band of connective tissue called the linea alba. Normally, this band is half an inch in width. Because of the action of relaxin, about 30 percent of all pregnant women experience an excessive loosening of this seam, a condition known as diastasis recti abdominis.

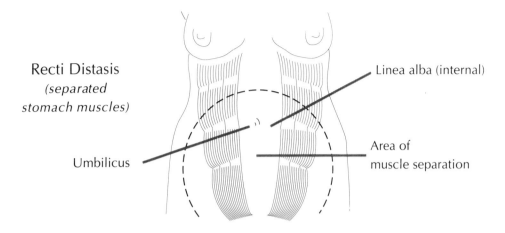

Recti Distasis
*(separated
stomach muscles)*

Linea alba (internal)

Umbilicus

Area of
muscle separation

MEASURING YOUR LINEA ALBA TISSUE

Before you do any exercise that impacts your abdomen, you'll want to measure the gap yourself to see if you are developing diastasis recti abdominis. Lie on your back and bend your knees toward your chest. Raise your head and shoulders very slightly by stretching your hands toward your feet. Feel for the separation in the area of your abdomen around your navel. If it is two or three finger widths or wider, women are advised against abdominal exercises, including leg lifts and sit-ups, which can increase the gap.

Hopefully, if you are aware of these muscle and skeletal changes that

MEASURING YOUR LINEA ALBA TISSUE

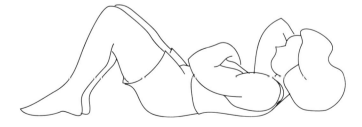

occur during pregnancy, you can modify your exercise patterns to accommodate these changes safely. Strengthening of the upper body and the abdominal muscles and practicing good posture are things that can be done before pregnancy and can help prevent, or alleviate, your discomforts in the coming months.

OVERHEATING

Most recommendations and guidelines about exercise during pregnancy warn against overheating. At Melpomene, we advise pregnant women to avoid exercising in hot environments and to be sure to take in enough fluids. The reasons for these recommendations are understandable if we consider the mechanisms for thermoregulation.

Your body has ingenious ways of getting rid of the heat you naturally generate. The heat is conducted outward to your skin and is dissipated as blood runs through the capillaries close to the surface. Your sweat glands provide a water-based cooling system. As sweat on your skin evaporates, it gives up heat, making you feel cooler in the process. During pregnancy heat is generated both by you and by the fetus. More blood is pumped to the skin, and more sweat is produced by the sweat glands. Sometimes, when the air outside the body is hot and humid, this cooling system can't work as efficiently, and both you and the fetus can become overheated.

Researchers working with animals know that maternal overheating early in gestation can cause defects in the fetus. We can't necessarily apply these studies to humans, however, because some of the animals have cooling mechanisms such as panting that are quite different from the mechanisms we use. Nevertheless, experts are convinced that the possible dangers of overheating are something to take into consideration, especially during exercise.

Of course, your temperature is bound to rise somewhat as you exercise. Keeping it within safe limits is the key. Robert Jones and colleagues at the Pennsylvania State University College of Medicine measured the core temperatures of four pregnant women before, during, and after they ran on a treadmill. All four women were runners before becoming pregnant and still ran regularly afterward. Their temperatures did increase during exercise and remained elevated for at least fifteen minutes after exercise. Temperature reduction to pre-exercise levels was especially slow during the third trimester. The researchers felt, however, that the temperature increases they saw were not dangerous. All the women went on to deliver healthy babies. While this study is reassuring, it is important to note that it involved only four women, and that these women were already accustomed to exercising. The length of time they exercised while their temperatures were measured was only twenty minutes.

Recently other scientists compared core temperatures of pregnant women who exercised for twenty minutes on a stationary bike when the bike was on dry land and when it was in water. Although temperature was affected in both mediums, it didn't rise quite as high in the women who biked in the water. If you live in a warm climate and want to exercise, you might be most comfortable if you choose water exercises. Once again, let your body be your guide.

Sometimes women wonder about the safety of hot tubs and saunas during pregnancy. Researchers who studied the medical histories of women with children who had birth defects did find a connection between raised temperatures and birth defects. In these cases, the mothers had either prolonged fevers during early pregnancy, or had spent long periods of time in hot tubs or saunas. These kinds of congenital problems are rare in Finland, however, where everyone takes saunas. A survey of the sauna habits of 100 pregnant Finnish women found that women who took saunas before pregnancy continued to do so when pregnant. There was a trend over the course of the nine months of pregnancy to shorten the length of time in the sauna and to lower the temperature of the sauna. Once again, common sense leads women to protect themselves. Studies show that most women, even when they are not pregnant, simply don't stay in uncomfortably hot saunas or hot tubs for dangerously long lengths of time. On the other hand, you may just want to avoid these two activities during your pregnancy.

So what can you do to avoid overheating?

1. Don't exercise in hot, humid environments. Sometimes an air-conditioned health club or a pool may be the best way to beat the heat in southern climes.

2. Drink more fluids. The more fluids you drink, the more freely you will perspire, and the cooler you'll be. Drinking enough fluids is also important during pregnancy to avoid dehydration, which has also been associated with premature labor. Don't *start* exercising if you feel particularly thirsty.

3. Do not exercise if you have a fever. Stop exercising if you are too warm. As with many other things during pregnancy, comfort is the key. There is no reason to subject yourself to any risk, no matter how minimal, by overheating. A shorter, less intense workout may be a wise choice on warm days. Everyone who exercises tries to minimize heat stress, and pregnant women should be no exception.

4. Keep the sauna or steam at a temperature at which you feel comfortable. This temperature may be far below your normal level of comfort, especially as your pregnancy progresses. Listen to your body!

EATING ENOUGH OF THE RIGHT FOODS

When women in the Melpomene study of exercise during pregnancy were asked if they had made any changes in their health habits during their pregnancies, the majority indicated they were trying to improve their dietary and eating patterns. Some were eating more protein. Many had increased the amounts of calcium-rich dairy products they ate. Others had cut out junk foods.

No research has been done on the nutritional requirements of physically active pregnant or breast-feeding women. According to Dr. Janet King, Melpomene advisory board member, we can only draw inferences from what we know about pregnant, sedentary women and nonpregnant, active women. We do know, for instance, that a woman's nutritional habits before and during pregnancy (and afterward if she is breast-feeding) are critical for the health of the mother and child. The mother's weight gain will affect the weight of the baby at birth; for example, heavier moms usually have heavier babies. Birth weights are important because low-weight babies are often at risk for health and developmental problems.

Despite the evidence that pregnant and breast-feeding women need proper nutrition, many women are still tempted to control their eating during this time. Because we've been imbued with the cultural ideal of female slenderness, many of us still feel anxious about the weight we are gaining, even if it is a normal and healthy amount. Many women put themselves on a strict diet throughout their pregnancy.

Conventional wisdom has long encouraged this behavior by telling pregnant women they should only gain a certain amount of weight during pregnancy. In western countries, this belief dates back to the eighteenth and nineteenth centuries when physicians thought they could make labor and delivery easier if babies were smaller at birth. Not only did they impose dietary controls on women to try to produce small babies but they even induced early labor.

After cesarean sections became available, there was less concern about the size of the baby and therefore fewer attempts to restrict diet and weight gain. But, as nutritionists Kathryn Dohrman and Sally Ledermann note, weight gain was blamed at the beginning of the twentieth century for a condition called toxemia. Toxemia is a general term used to describe disorders of late pregnancy in which hypertension, proteinuria (protein in the urine), and edema (fluid retention) occur. Convulsions and coma may also be associated with toxemia. Experts mistakenly believed that weight gain caused toxemia, when in reality, it was the other way around. Toxemia caused weight gain through fluid retention! At the same time, scientists developed the mistaken theory that the fetus is a perfect parasite whose nutritional needs would always be met by the mother's stores or intake. Thus, women began to restrict their diets to prevent toxemia, thinking that the fetus would just naturally adjust to the lower food intake.

Today, although we know better, women are still restricting their diets, this time for different reasons. The myth that says women have to be thin to be attractive is alive and well, and larger women, pregnant or not, are seen as lacking self-control. Despite the fact that it can be detrimental to mother and baby, dieting during pregnancy is culturally endorsed.

Thus, many women are searching for a guideline for how much they are "allowed" to eat, because unfortunately, most adult women in the

United States are not in the habit of simply eating when they are hungry. There is no such thing as a "best" weight gain during pregnancy—that depends entirely on you, the individual. Factors to be considered include your pre-pregnancy weight and your level of physical activity. If you are thin, you may need to gain more than a heavier woman. If you are physically active, you'll need to eat enough to cover the cost of fetal growth, added maternal tissue, and the energy needed for physical activity.

Keep in mind that pregnancy itself is bound to change your eating habits, especially when physical changes begin to affect your appetite. For example, morning sickness early in pregnancy, which may be due to high levels of chorionic gonadotropin hormone, will make crackers look more attractive than steak.

Some of the unpleasant side effects of pregnancy, such as nausea, heartburn, indigestion, and constipation, are caused by an increase in a steroid called progesterone. Progesterone causes the smooth muscles of the gastrointestinal tract to relax so that food moves through the stomach and bowels more slowly, resulting in the feeling of fullness, heartburn, or nausea. Slower movement in the gut also means more water is absorbed by the intestines—a probable cause of constipation. Exercise is often recommended as a way to promote regularity, and the pregnant women in our study vouched for its effectiveness.

Progesterone is also responsible for an increase in appetite felt by pregnant women. (Yes, it's true that you really might feel hungrier when you are pregnant!) But as pregnancy progresses and the uterus begins to displace other internal organs, you may prefer to eat several small meals rather than a few large meals. Much of what you eat will be converted into fatty deposits in your hips, thighs, and abdomen, especially during the second trimester. This fat deposition is your body's preparation for lactation and is a predictable outcome of increased progesterone.

Of course, when you're interested in good nutrition, it's not only the quantity of food taken in (the total number of calories) that is important but also the quality of the diet. Research shows that some pregnant women can maintain their weight even at very low intake levels. The mechanism for this maintenance is not known. It may be that a pregnant woman's metabolism becomes more efficient, allowing her to maintain her weight. It may also be that pregnant women instinctively decrease their level of activity and therefore save energy. We know from our research that recreational athletes tend to voluntarily reduce their exercise activity over the three trimesters of their pregnancy.

The body seems to be well-adapted to make the most of what you feed it during pregnancy. But again, the question arises, "What if you add exercise to the equation? Will that change your nutritional needs?" Melpomene has the only data available on the nutritional habits of physically active pregnant and breast-feeding women. Based on diet histories and activity logs we found that pregnant women runners:

- Consumed fewer calories than what would normally be required by their level of physical activity.
- Had diets that were low in iron and calcium (below RDA standards).

And yet these women were maintaining their weight, perhaps through some of the mechanisms we mentioned above. The deficiency in iron in their diets might have been a problem, but most of the women were also taking iron supplements to compensate for what they lacked in their diets. Anemia is common in pregnancy because there is an increase in blood volume (the total amount of blood) without an equivalent rise in red blood cells. In terms of calcium, it appears that metabolic and physiologic changes help the body actually conserve calcium during pregnancy. In general, for women who were getting enough calcium in their pre-pregnancy diets, supplements during pregnancy do not seem to make much difference. However, our diet logs show that most women do not meet recommended daily allowance (RDA) requirements in their normal diets, so we usually suggest that they increase their calcium intake.

We do not yet have enough information to know whether there are specific nutrient needs for pregnant women who exercise. To be on the safe side, you'd be wise to make sure your diet is high in vitamins and minerals. Whether you are pregnant or not, good diets are always preferable to using dietary supplements.

GUIDELINES FOR EXERCISE DURING PREGNANCY

*Stay within your body's limits—it will "tell" you to back
off if problems arise.*
—MICHELE DAVIS, A NATIONALLY RANKED WOMAN RUNNER WHO RAN IN
THE OLYMPIC MARATHON TRIALS DURING ONE OF HER TWO "RUNNING"
PREGNANCIES.

There are many sets of guidelines for women wishing to exercise during pregnancy. The American College of Obstetrics and Gynecology has issued one set, which physicians frequently use. We at Melpomene have our own recommendations based specifically on the research we have done. Remember that for many sports there are only anecdotal reports and little or no direct research data available from which to compose guidelines. Because we have worked primarily with pregnant runners and swimmers and with maternal fitness programs, our guidelines refer to these activities only.

We'll begin with general guidelines for anyone considering exercise while pregnant. Also, we strongly encourage you to seek out guidelines that would speak to your own unique medical history. Say, for instance, you have gestational diabetes. You would then be most interested in a recent booklet published by the International Diabetes Center on gestational diabetes. Nutritionist Marion Franz and her associates believe that exercise is important for diabetic women because it can help keep blood glucose at normal levels. They recommend taking a walk after breakfast, when blood sugars tend to be elevated. If you are aware of such a condition in your medical history, you may want to contact the association that distributes information and conducts research on that condition. Ask your healthcare provider where to find these resources.

GENERAL GUIDELINES

1. Discuss your exercise plans with your healthcare provider, especially if medical conditions might present problems, for example, history of miscarriage.
2. Find out about special guidelines that may pertain to your own medical condition. Say you had gestational diabetes. A booklet put out by the International Diabetes Center recommends exercise as a way to keep blood glucose levels at normal levels. Ask your healthcare provider about agencies or nonprofit groups that may distribute information on your condition.
3. Get support for your decision to exercise or not to exercise from friends, your spouse, and even your physician.
4. Wear comfortable clothing. Well-cushioned stable shoes and a good bra are important.
5. Listen to your body. "No pain, no gain" does not apply to exercising during pregnancy.
6. Expect some discomfort. Learn all you can about exercising during pregnancy in order to have examples of how much discomfort is ordinary and what may be reason for concern.
7. Be flexible. Do not have preset goals for exercising during pregnancy. Avoid excessive competition, so you can go at your own pace. Be prepared to stop or switch to another form of exercise if you experience discomfort or fatigue.
8. Stop exercising and check with your instructor and/or healthcare provider if you have any questions about your health or change in your condition. Seek immediate advice if you have pain, dizziness, light-headedness, sudden confusion, lack of coordination, nausea or vomiting, vaginal bleeding, breathlessness lasting more than ten minutes, rapid heart rate ten minutes after aerobic exercise, or prolonged fatigue.
9. Be alert to changing conditions in your pregnancy, which may call for you to change or stop your exercise, such as early thinning (effacement) or opening (dilation) of the cervix, or finding out you are pregnant with twins.
10. Avoid an anaerobic (breathless) pace.

11. Avoid overheating and dehydration. Drink plenty of fluids before, during, and after your exercise routine.
12. Avoid injury to joints and ligaments. Take the time to adequately warm up and cool down. Avoid stretching to the point of maximum resistance. Pay attention to your balance and posture.
13. Be sure to get adequate rest. Exercising to the point of exhaustion or chronic fatigue is detrimental to both mother and fetus.
14. Be sure to meet your nutritional needs. Your diet should provide the extra energy you need for exercise, as well as the nutritional foundation for pregnancy itself. A healthy weight gain is a good indicator that you are eating enough. Iron and calcium supplements, which are normally recommended to pregnant women, are also important.
15. Once you start, stay in the habit of exercising. Exercise twenty to thirty minutes at least three times a week, preferably on alternate days. Irregular or infrequent exercise can lead to injury and fatigue.

HOW TO EVALUATE MATERNAL FITNESS PROGRAMS

Maternal fitness programs have become quite popular in recent years, and there are a number of classes to choose from, including some that are available on videocassette. No thorough, independent evaluation of any of these programs has yet been done. The best we can do is offer you some help in selecting a program that you feel will be safe and effective for you.

Before you begin a maternal fitness program, we suggest you consult your doctor or midwife. Discuss your exercise needs in light of your medical history and your current physical condition. Get medical approval before you begin. Then select a sound exercise program with a qualified instructor. *Be choosy.*

At the heart of a good exercise program is a well-qualified instructor. Look for an instructor:

- Who is sensitive to the health education needs of pregnant women.
- Who has an extensive background as an exercise instructor.
- Who has training that includes information specific to pregnancy and childbirth.

- Who will assess and monitor your health and fitness level, modifying the exercise program to reflect your needs.
- Who will teach you to identify signs and symptoms of potential problems, ways to reduce the risk of injury, how to monitor your heart rate, and the importance of fluid replacement.

In addition to a well-qualified instructor, a good prenatal exercise program will have the following basic components:

1. *Warm-up period* to protect joints and muscles from injury and to slowly increase breathing and heart rates.
2. *Muscle strengthening exercises* to build and maintain tone and strength.
3. *Cardiovascular conditioning exercises* to build and maintain heart and lung strength and endurance. *Note:* The American College of Obstetricians and Gynecologists recommends that your heart rate not exceed 140 beats per minute.
4. *Cool-down period* to safely ease breathing and heart rates to a lower level of activity.
5. *Relaxation techniques* to identify and release muscle tension and help metabolism return to normal.
6. *Health education and discussion period* to foster a supportive atmosphere for the discussion of concerns related to pregnancy.

CHECKLIST FOR EVALUATING AN EXERCISE PROGRAM
DURING PREGNANCY

Call several programs to determine which ones could meet your needs. You can ask:

What are the goals of the exercise program? How do you evaluate whether these goals are being met?

Describe a typical class session from beginning to end.

Are participants required to check their heart rates and drink fluids?

What are the qualifications of the instructor?

Is a medical permit and/or medical history required of participants?

What is the maximum class size?
Is there an opportunity to evaluate the program and the instructor?
What is the cost of the program? Are scholarships available?
What is the registration procedure?
Are potential participants permitted to observe the class?
Is a postnatal program offered?
Is childcare available? What is the cost?
What is the availability of medical help if there is an emergency?

Select one or two programs and ask permission to observe a class. Meet with the instructor and talk with class members. Choose the program that best meets your needs.

Once you begin, keep exercising. Regular exercise can increase your flexibility while strengthening your heart and lungs, bones, and muscles. Now that you have established an exercise habit, keep it up for life!

RECOMMENDATIONS FOR RUNNERS WHO WISH TO EXERCISE DURING PREGNANCY

1. Overheating or not drinking enough can cause serious problems. Run in the coolest part of the day and in appropriate clothing. Be sure to drink plenty of fluids before a run—even if you may have to stop for bathroom breaks more often.
2. Take the time for adequate warm-up and cool-down before and after running.
3. Wear comfortable clothing. Well-cushioned stable running shoes and a good bra are important.
4. Some women find a lightweight maternity girdle offers support for back and ligaments. Maternity support stockings also help some women feel more comfortable.
5. Be willing to modify your runs in terms of intensity, frequency, and speed. Increasing weight and fatigue may dictate shorter, slower runs, eliminating hills and speed work.
6. Stop and walk if necessary. You may feel a need to slow down because of heat, ligament or joint pains, Braxton-Hicks contractions (incidental contractions, not related to labor), and so forth.

7. Run with others, if possible. Always let people know when and where you are running. Bring money in case you need to phone someone to take you home.
8. Be kind to your back. Pay attention to your posture and balance. You may want to experiment with posture changes that make you more stable while running.
9. Modify or stop your exercise program if medical conditions dictate, for example, early dilation or bag of waters leaking.

Nurse and runner, Annemarie Jutel, has given some thought to the kinds of specific problems pregnant runners might face and possible solutions. Among the things she mentions are rest as the appropriate response to fatigue, nausea, and shortness of breath. Remember that it is natural to feel more tired, given the increased cost of weight-bearing exercise as your body weight increases. To avoid an anaerobic pace, try short wind sprints if you still want to have a chance to run fast. All of these suggestions underscore the importance of remaining flexible in your exercise habits and paying close attention to your body.

RECOMMENDATIONS FOR SWIMMERS WHO WISH TO EXERCISE DURING PREGNANCY

1. Be sure the water and air temperatures are comfortable. Leave the water if you feel uncomfortably chilly or overheated.
2. Take time to warm up. Try doing some stretching on land or in the water. Start off swimming slowly until you loosen up.
3. Wear a comfortable suit. Some maternity suits may be too heavy when wet for easy swimming. Experiment with different fabrics, styles, and sizes until you find something that gives you support where you need it and in which you can swim well.
4. Swim according to your abilities. Use moderation and be sure to breathe properly.
5. Avoid diving, jumping into the water feet first, and water skiing while you are pregnant.
6. If you experience contractions, leg cramps, or joint pain, be ready to

stop swimming, or change your swimming style, for example, use different strokes, kicks, or turns.
7. Do not swim alone, but do try to avoid crowds.
8. Modify or stop your exercise program if medical conditions dictate, for example, early dilation or bag of waters leaking.

LABOR AND DELIVERY

Various historical sources, including the Bible, infer that an active pregnancy is apt to make for an easier labor and delivery. Research data to support these suggestions are not as clear. Some researchers have suggested that female athletes might have more difficulty with labor and delivery because of their "overly" developed musculature. Others believe just the opposite.

Gyula Erdelyi, one of the earliest researchers, presented a paper on the medical aspects of sports in 1960. He reported that Olympic-caliber women athletes had easy deliveries with short second stages and few cesarean sections. More recent studies of women with first-time pregnancies showed that those who took part in the strength training and aerobic maternal fitness programs also had a lower-than-average number of cesarean sections, but their labors were of average length. A third set of results comes from Pat Kulpa, an obstetrician/gynecologist in Washington, who studied women who engaged in regular aerobic exercise and some who did not. Dr. Kulpa and her colleagues found that for first-time mothers, there was no difference in cesarean section rates between the exercising and nonexercising women.

Another conflict in results occurred when researchers examined whether or not exercise puts women at risk for premature births. In Vermont, Dr. Clapp found that women who exercised aerobically into the third trimester not only gained less weight and had lighter babies but also delivered their babies earlier than women who had stopped exercising earlier. It is important to note that this association between gestational length, maternal weight gain, and birth weight with exercise has not been duplicated by other researchers. In fact, a study in Oregon showed that all of the seventeen women who exercised during their third trimester had normal, forty-week gestations with no increase in premature uterine contractions. Their labors and deliveries were normal, and their babies were healthy.

The conflicts in findings about exercise, labor, and delivery reflect some of the problems in coming to uniform conclusions about possible benefits as well as problems of exercising while pregnant. It is hard to predict the course of labor because each woman's experience is as individual as she is. Exercise, being only one variable, may not play the deciding role.

POSTPARTUM CONSIDERATIONS

While researchers struggle with the question of whether or not exercise is safe during pregnancy, women continue to get pregnant and invariably some continue to exercise. After their babies are born, they wonder about resuming exercise, and about regaining their pre-pregnancy level of activity and fitness.

Recently the media has played up the postpregnancy athletic performances of a few elite women. Suddenly there is talk of the "training effect of pregnancy." In an absurd leap, we have moved from wondering whether we should exercise during pregnancy to recommending pregnancy as a way to improve athletic ability. Aside from the anecdotal accounts of people like Ingrid Kristiansen and Mary Decker Slaney, however, there is not much data to back up this kind of recommendation.

Most women are usually advised to wait four or six weeks after an uncomplicated vaginal delivery before they start exercising again. In Melpomene's research, and from our conversations with physically active women, we know that many women do not wait this long. Therefore, we decided to include a list of commonsense considerations for women who want to exercise during the immediate postpartum period. Look for them at the end of this section, on page 140.

In general, you'll want to keep in mind that your body took nine months to change, and that those changes aren't about to reverse themselves overnight. For example, relaxin softened your connective tissues so they could stretch to accommodate the growing fetus and the pressures of labor and delivery. One place this occurred was in the pelvic floor, where the muscles that hold together your internal organs are found. The fascia that connect these muscles stretched during pregnancy, and once stretched, fascia will never regain their former shape. To compensate for the loss of support, you may want to work on strengthening your muscles in this area as well as others.

Kegel exercises are often recommended for strengthening the muscles in the pelvic floor (see page 164). These exercises may also help lessen the problem of urinary incontinence that many women experience after delivery, especially during weight-bearing activities such as running.

Finding time to exercise is a lesson in creative time management for the new mother. If she chooses to breast-feed (as did more than 90 percent of the women in Melpomene's studies of exercise and pregnancy), there will be additional constraints in scheduling. We advise women to feed first, then exercise to avoid the discomfort of overly full breasts. For the first few months, however, arranging childcare to meet a baby's changing schedule may be as stressful an exercise as you can manage!

Besides practical problems like childcare, breast-feeding women are also concerned about nutrition. While women want to eat and drink enough to maintain a good milk supply, many are eager to return to a lower weight. In our research, we found that women tend to greatly increase their exercise level in postpartum, while eating fewer calories than they did during pregnancy. Many asked us, "Is it all right to be losing weight while I'm breast-feeding? Is the baby getting all the nutrients needed for growth?" Overall, we feel that infant weight gain, not maternal weight loss, should be used as the measure of appropriate maternal diet by breast-feeding women.

As we have seen in many other facets of childbearing, the female body is superbly designed for reproduction. While you are breast-feeding, your body won't let you lose weight too quickly. Breast-feeding slows the rate of weight loss, perhaps as a way to conserve resources for the baby. Eventually, the breast-feeding women in our study did lose all the weight they had gained, but it took them between three and nine months after the birth. The women who were not breast-feeding lost it faster, but they also tended to be more active and to eat less.

Some researchers have expressed concern about the relation between breast-feeding and osteoporosis, the thinning of the bones that is a major health concern for women (see discussion on page 169). The average woman in this country does not get enough calcium in her diet, and according to Melpomene's pregnancy study results, this is also true for most women who exercise during pregnancy and while breast-feeding.

A recent study by Gary Chan at the University of Utah medical center found that sedentary women who breast-fed for more than six months showed bone loss even though they had calcium intakes above the RDA. How might these women have fared if they had been exercising? Recent evidence points to the fact that exercise may actually increase bone mass. It will be important for researchers to explore the relationship between exercise, calcium intake, bone mass, and breast-feeding.

Another postpartum reality for many new mothers is depression, fatigue, and a feeling of being overwhelmed by their new role. At two months postpartum, about half of all the women in Melpomene's study perceived themselves to have experienced the "postpartum blues." This depression hit both the exercising and the nonexercising women. One woman recalled, "During the first week I was very tired and I couldn't stop crying." At this point, we do not know enough about the possible influence of exercise on postpartum depression.

When asked if they felt fully recovered, or back to "being themselves" after two months, only 53 percent of the runners, 60 percent of the swimmers, and 50 percent of the sedentary women answered yes. Whether this response refers to mental or physical recovery we do not know. All but one woman in the study did report herself to be in good or excellent health. Many may still have been trying to recapture pre-pregnancy activity levels and/or weight. To all new mothers, we say "Try not to be impatient. Postpartum is the rest of your life!"

EXERCISING AFTER YOUR BABY IS BORN

After the birth of the baby, most women are eager to resume pre-pregnancy activities, including exercise. Many come to us for guidelines or precautions. Unfortunately, we have little hard data, because very little research has been done on women who resume exercise after delivery. What we do pass along is information we have gleaned from the participants in our exercise and pregnancy research.

The first step is to discuss your exercise plan with your healthcare provider. If you've had a cesarean section, it is especially important to consider your physician's instructions.

If you had an uncomplicated vaginal delivery, we suggest you consider these points before you start exercising:

1. If you had an episiotomy, you will probably want to wait until all soreness is gone before you exercise vigorously.
2. Since you cannot use tampons for about four weeks, you may find it more convenient to wait until bleeding has stopped.
3. If you exercise and begin to bleed heavily, and/or with bright red blood, you should give yourself more time to recover.
4. Since your hormonal balance does not stabilize for several weeks, be aware of continuing joint laxity (looseness).
5. Fatigue is a common problem for new mothers. If you are tired, it might be better to take a nap than to exercise. This suggestion is especially true if you are nursing.
6. Nursing mothers should remember to drink lots of fluids.
7. For women who are breast-feeding, good breast support during exercise is important.
8. Often, women are surprised to find they are incontinent after delivery. This problem can last for several months. The best exercises to correct this condition are Kegel's (see page 164).
9. Sometimes the cumulative effects of pregnancy, labor, and carrying a baby lead to back pain. Watch your posture. Doing some abdominal strengthening exercises may help (see precautions on page 123).
10. Take time to warm up and stretch before exercise, and give yourself an ample cool-down and relaxation period after exercise.
11. Be sure to practice good nutritional habits. Though it may be inconvenient to eat properly when you have a baby and a busy schedule, it's worth the effort. There is also no reason to rush into weight loss, especially if you are nursing. Breast-feeding women lose weight more slowly because of the body's protective mechanisms.
12. Scheduling will take some juggling. Many women find it is difficult

to make childcare arrangements and/or find the time to exercise in the early months.

13. Relax and enjoy yourself! A brisk walk with your baby may be all you can do at first. As you develop a routine and can fit in regular exercise, you will find it provides important time for yourself.

Attitudes toward women and their body are changing. Pregnancy is no longer viewed as a diseased state or a time when women are expected to be incapacitated. Few women take to their beds when they become pregnant; instead, many are simply buying a larger pair of workout clothes and continuing to exercise.

Research by obstetrician/gynecologist Pat Kulpa has shown that cardiovascular fitness can actually be improved by exercising while you're pregnant. Even so, many of the specific questions relating to physiology and the effects of exercise during pregnancy have yet to be answered. If you're pregnant today, you may feel as if you can't wait until science has all the answers.

The decisions you make about your lifestyle during pregnancy are personal ones. Because of our society's emphasis on fitness, you may feel as much pressure to exercise during pregnancy as not to exercise. As a pregnant woman, you naturally feel a responsibility to your unborn child and you need support for your decisions and actions. At Melpomene, we encourage women to take an active role in managing their pregnancy. We know, however, that not everything can be controlled. No one can guarantee a perfect pregnancy, or a wished-for pregnancy outcome. No matter how carefully you try to make healthy choices, the unexpected can happen. Remember that exercise is only one of many variables, known and unknown, that can influence the course of a pregnancy.

Over and over again, women have told us that exercise helped make their pregnancies enjoyable. Many women have also told us that the questions and adjustments they made in their physical activity during pregnancy helped them remember how to enjoy exercise. Pregnancy is a time to think about priorities. We hope that the steps you take to ensure a healthy pregnancy are steps that will lead you to a healthy lifestyle long after your baby is born.

AN IRON FAMILY PORTRAIT

By the time he was born on April 22, 1988, Blaine Bradley Limberg had completed four triathlons, a biathlon, and a cross-country ski race. One of the triathlons included the World Championship Hawaii Ironman, a grueling event for anyone, which includes a 2-mile ocean swim, a 110-mile bike ride, and a 26.2-mile marathon run. Blaine's mom, athlete Barb Bradley, completed the Ironman when she was three and a half months pregnant.

According to Barb, the pregnancy was a surprise. A competitive athlete all her life, Barb was training hard to qualify for the Ironman. A pregnancy test explained her fatigue and stomach pains. Her first thoughts, of course, were to ensure the health of her baby and herself. She wondered if she could do this and still compete in the Ironman.

Barb and her husband, Allen Limberg (who was also training for the Ironman), began to seek "objective information—not subjective advice." After consulting the midwives and ob/gyn managing her pregnancy, as well as others who had information about exercise and pregnancy, Barb decided that in her training and competing she would be especially careful in three areas:

1. *Temperature.* She wanted to keep her core temperature below 101°F.
2. *Drinking plenty of fluids.* Urinating every two to three hours was Barb's way of being sure she was taking in enough fluids.
3. *Fatigue.* One of the things Barb did to avoid fatigue was to cut back her training by about half. Barb says this decision was a personal, subjective one and was not based on any specific recommendations.

Barb also stayed alert to anything unusual or abnormal in the way she felt.

Overall, Barb had an easy pregnancy. She remembers that she did feel like she was "training at altitude" and experienced some shortness of breath and fatigue. Overall, the training was successful, and Barb and her husband decided that if things were going well, she would enter the Ironman.

What was it like to be pregnant and in the Ironman? Race day was very emotional. Barb had decided to approach the race with the attitude, "I'm not a competitor. I'm a participant." As she stood on the starting line, she felt cautious, yet confident. The Labman medical group, which tests a range of athletes during the race, had given her a prerace ultrasound, and had agreed to monitor her temperature throughout the day. Before her pregnancy, Barb's goal had been to complete the Ironman in 12 hours. By taking it easy, she was able to finish in 14.5 hours, yet she never pushed herself beyond what was comfortable for her or her baby. The Labman group found she had actually gained a pound during the race by drinking large amounts of fluids frequently. Her postrace ultrasound showed all was well.

Barb's 7-pound 3-ounce and 20-inch son Blaine was born after a thirty-three hour labor. Barb actually rode her bike seventeen miles on the day she went into labor. Within two weeks of delivery she was back on her bike and by three months she was back to her normal routine.

What advice would this Ironmom give to other women wondering about exercise and pregnancy?

1. Consider your health.
2. Consider your baby's health.
3. Consider your exercise background.
4. Monitor yourself.
5. Know yourself.

Barb believes, as did many of the women in Melpomene's exercise and pregnancy studies, that the major benefits of exercise are the same during pregnancy as they are at any time, and for anyone. It makes you feel good psychologically and physically. During pregnancy, exercise also helps maintain a good body image because it gives women a sense of control over their bodies at a time when there are so many uncontrollable physical changes occurring.

Wisely, Barb does not want her experience to be used to push women to exercise during pregnancy, but she does want other women to know what can be done.

F I V E

RAISING YOUR CHILD TO BE ACTIVE

Our doctors, our health officials, and even our entertainers have become evangelical in recent years about the benefits of a physically active lifestyle. By now, most adults are aware of the many good reasons they should tear themselves away from TV and start to exercise: weight control, improved appearance, greater capacity and endurance for work and recreation, reduced stress, socializing opportunities, and generally enhanced well-being. But how many adults think about the benefits their children might gain through regular exercise, recreation, and sport? How many parents consider it their responsibility to encourage and facilitate physical activity for their kids?

But aren't children active enough? Many of us have vivid memories of an active childhood—long days of running, biking, swimming, and playing kickball in the schoolyard. We assume that children today must also get enough exercise in their normal patterns of play. Some kids do in fact stay fit by playing and participating in family recreation or organized sports. However, recent studies are showing that a significant number of children are spending their long days in front of a TV or video monitor, or in equally passive activities.

A growing number of health fitness professionals, teachers, coaches, and parents are concerned about this sedentary "couch potato" lifestyle. While many adults are meeting the challenge to become more physically fit, too many children and adolescents are steering away from active pursuits such as swimming, hiking, bicycling, sports teams, skiing, and the myriad other physical activities available.

Several national studies have tracked this trend over the past two decades:

- In 1984, the National Children and Youth Fitness Study discovered that only half of the 8,800 fifth through twelfth graders surveyed were getting the minimum amount of year-round physical activity needed to maintain cardiorespiratory capacity.
- The Health and Nutrition Examination Surveys, which periodically measure children's health and nutritional status, documented a significant rise in obesity over the past twenty years.
- The 1985 President's Council on Physical Fitness and Sports Study indicated that U.S. schoolchildren are performing lower than in recent years on standard tests for endurance, strength, and flexibility. This study also found that a significant proportion of children have one or more heart disease risk factors, namely high blood pressure, high blood cholesterol levels, or obesity.
- In the 1970s, Gilliam and fellow researchers reported similar findings in their study of heart disease risk factors in seven- to twelve-year-olds. A study of Muscatine, Iowa, schoolchildren by Lauer had more of the same bad news.

Obviously, it's not enough for us to rely on children's so-called natural inclination toward physical activity. Simply being "a kid" does not automatically make your child physically fit, nor will it prevent or reduce the risk that he or she will develop heart disease as an adult. Regular exercise can help minimize these risk factors, however, and with luck, can trigger a healthy habit that will continue into adulthood.

As a parent, how can you tell whether your child is physically fit? In 1987, we asked mothers to describe their children's fitness, and received responses ranging from "she has a thin, frail body type and no interest in athletics," and "he prefers not to work hard or sweat," to "he is agile, fast, energetic, just the right weight, and looks trim," and "she has very good coordination and is in the President's Council on Physical Fitness and Sports Program for five-year-olds."

In reality, physical fitness can be difficult to measure, especially in growing children. Part of the difficulty lies in deciding which of the fitness parameters to include in the definition. Endurance, flexibility, athletic skills, work capacity, resistance to illness, body type, muscle mass, weight, body fat, and capacity to deal with physical and emotional stress are all valid indicators of fitness. Although researchers and educators differ on the particulars of fitness assessment, most agree that all children should be exercising or involved in recreational or sports activities, each to his or her own physical potential.

How, then, do you as a parent help your child get involved in and excited about physical activity? What if you and your spouse or partner have not yet made exercise a regular part of your life? How do you figure out what will motivate your child?

At the Melpomene Institute, we are as curious as you are. In 1986, we started a long-term national study tracking the physical activity patterns of children from early childhood through adolescence. We used questionnaires to find out (1) what motivates children to participate in recreation and sports, and (2) what factors are most critical in establishing a lifelong pattern of physical activity. We were able to get some generational data because many of the moms who responded are women who participated in our exercise and pregnancy studies. The two family profiles below represent the range of physical activity patterns documented through the first surveys conducted in 1986 through 1988. As you read them, think of how the members in your own family prefer to spend their time.

PROFILES OF TWO FAMILIES

Mark and Timmy are brothers who get along well despite their age difference. Mark is nine and his little brother just turned five. Both boys are bright and interested in the world around them. Their parents are continually helping them learn by reading to them and taking them to museums and the planetarium. The time Mark and Timmy spend with their parents is treasured by all since both parents are busy with their teaching jobs and volunteer committee and board activities.

Neither one of the boys has pursued many physical or recreational activities so far. Mark tried swimming lessons the summer he turned six, but he didn't care for the water and hasn't been swimming much since. He does ride his bike with his friends, but they don't often venture beyond their neighborhood park, where they spend most of their time making up detective and spy stories and playacting horror shows—great fun, but not very active. Mark spends most of his remaining free time conducting experiments for his science club.

Timmy is sometimes allowed to join the older boys, but he usually spends time with his neighbor friends Billy and Elizabeth, playing the educational games his parents give him or a variety of imaginary games. Timmy spends weekdays in daycare, and although there are scheduled opportunities for playing on the jungle gym and swimming, Timmy shies away from these activities, preferring to draw and color. His parents believe he is very artistic and they encourage him to develop that interest.

The boys' parents have never been athletically inclined, and with so many other interests, they haven't shared many recreational activities with their children. They do not have any particularly negative feelings toward physical activity, but they do not consider it an integral or necessary part of their lifestyle. Both mom and dad think their boys have enough other activities to keep them busy, and the boys don't complain that they are missing out on anything.

Becky and Jeff are both active youngsters. At ten, Becky is proud of her gymnastics skills. She's been involved in gymnastics all her life, beginning with the Babygym class her mother brought her to when she was two and a half. Becky loves to try new stunts and has developed strong leg and arm muscles. She has also taken swimming lessons for several years and recently began studying karate after visiting some of the classes her father teaches. Becky has been to summer camp for three consecutive years and thoroughly enjoys the lake swimming and canoe outings. Becky spends the remainder of her leisure time practicing piano. She is very musical and enjoys being in recitals.

Seven-year-old Jeff is not as strong for his age, but he has always tried to keep up with his older sister, as well as his parents. Ever since he could walk, Jeff has joined his mother on the community fun runs and walks for parents and children. He loves to run and just finished his first children's one-kilometer race. Mom enjoys taking Jeff along when she jogs around the neighborhood. She invites Becky to join them, but Becky doesn't care for running, so her mom doesn't push it. Jeff also enjoys being on a T-ball team and playing catch with his sister. At other times, Jeff works on his nature book, collecting and drawing plant specimens.

Both parents grew up participating in a host of outdoor and sports activities, and they enjoy sharing those interests with Becky and Jeff. The family takes frequent camping trips that include lots of hiking and canoeing. In the winter they switch to cross-country skiing and snowshoeing. In both settings the parents try to make these outings enjoyable learning experiences by teaching Becky and Jeff about nature, wildlife, and respect for the outdoors. They also prefer to emphasize fun and building self-confidence rather than competition and skilled athletic training.

Both mom and dad work, so they agree that these shared recreational outings contribute to making a closer family. They have always enrolled Becky and Jeff in a variety of sports lessons, but have never forced them to continue any activity in which they've had little interest or ability. Both parents believe it's important to expose their children to lots of activities, let the kids choose their favorites, and then do everything they can to encourage those choices.

CHILDREN'S PHYSICAL ACTIVITY PATTERNS: HOW ARE THEY INFLUENCED?

According to our most recent survey of mothers across the country, one-fifth of their one- to thirteen-year-old children were more like Mark and Timmy—not very active. One-third of the boys and girls were moderately active, and more encouraging, nearly half were very active. (To determine whether children were very active, moderately active, or not very active, we asked mothers how many physical activities their children had participated in over their lifetimes, how often they participated, and at what ages they began those activities.)

Why is there such a disparity in activity levels for these children? What contributes to making some girls and boys so much more active than their counterparts? It appears from the Melpomene study as well as from other research that the combined influence of family, community, and school contribute significantly to whether and how extensively children become and remain physically active.

John Thatcher, the director of sports medicine at East Stroudsburg University in Pennsylvania, concludes that parents can exert a very posi-

tive influence on their children's physical activity and fitness levels by
letting their children see how much mom and dad enjoy being active and
by asking their children to join them in recreational and sports activities.
As parents in the Melpomene studies begin to tell us their stories, we can
also see how instrumental parents' own activities can be in spurring young
children's interest:

> "Our family is active. The kids and my husband and I watch little or
> no television. We are not pushing our kids into organized sports or
> classes, but are letting them play on their own and with us. This year
> we plan to begin our seven-year-old on downhill skiing."

> "When the weather is warm I take the kids running with me . . . I
> push two strollers . . . I call it "quality running." It must have some
> influence on them—I sometimes catch them putting their stuffed an-
> imals in the stroller and running behind, telling me they're "out jog-
> ging." My three-and-a-half-year-old son does push-ups like Mom and
> Dad. As the kids grow, we will let them know what physical activities
> are out there, but it will be up to them as to what they want to
> pursue."

> "Compared to other children their age, our boys both run faster and
> last longer . . . Both my husband and I enjoy outdoors and physical
> activity, so the kids model us and participate with us in many activ-
> ities."

> "Our four-year-old daughter is very active and always running. She
> tells Mom that she wants to run in races like she does."

> "My two-and-a-half-year-old daughter walks with me to do errands.
> She also plays outside with me a lot and jogs one block at a time with
> me. She is very physically fit for her age."

> "My three-year-old son likes to imitate his mom. He goes with me on
> lots of training runs and rides."

Beyond the narratives, the numerical survey results show that these parents' attitudes toward physical activity are likely to influence their children's perceptions. In our 1987 survey, we found that children who had more physically active mothers also had higher physical activity levels. We asked all mothers to rate how much of an impact, if any, various factors had on their child's participation in physical activities and sports. The twenty-one factors were drawn from psychological, social, and environmental variables identified in behavioral and health education research. These factors included mothers' and fathers' activity patterns and expectations, siblings' activity patterns, school and recreational physical activity programs, competing leisure time activities, and the child's physical status and abilities.

The most highly ranked positive influences were mothers' and fathers' own physical activity patterns. Children who see their parents jog in the neighborhood, ride their bikes for transportation and recreation, or hear about how much they enjoy their tennis matches or cross-country ski trips tend to get a positive image of physical activity. Next to role modeling, the second most positive influence was the time both mothers and fathers spend with their children doing physical activities. Being active with their moms and dads seems to have a very positive influence on the youngsters' overall participation in exercise, recreation, and sports.

Factors outside the home were also found to be significant positive influences on children's involvement in physical activities. Most notable were community recreation programs, sports lessons and classes, extracurricular school sports programs, and access to recreational facilities such as parks and swimming pools. Parents play a valuable role here, too, by finding out what programs and facilities are available, discussing their children's interests, encouraging them to participate, and taking an ongoing interest in their experiences with these activities.

Other variables also have important, positive influences on children's sports and recreation patterns. As might be expected, children with good overall health and good athletic skills are more inclined to be physically active. However, many parents who responded to our surveys said their children had substantial interest in physical activities despite their small size, lagging muscle development, or lack of physical abilities. If a child has a risk-taking or assertive personality, or if his or her parents strongly reinforce each achievement, the child can often overcome disadvantages in physical stature or skill. Parents' expectations for their children's achievements in sports or recreational activities can also positively influence the children's desires to attempt and stick to activities, provided those expectations are reasonable and do not make excessive demands on their children, either physically or emotionally.

WHAT CAN CHILDREN DO TO BECOME PHYSICALLY ACTIVE?

In our 1987 survey, we asked parents to list the number of physical activities in which their child had ever participated. Some parents were unable to name even one, whereas others listed fifteen. The average was five activities. The average age children began their first activity was just over sixteen months, and on average, the children had tried two physical activities by the time they were three years old.

The most popular activity was swimming lessons; fully two-thirds of the children who had participated in at least one physical activity had taken swimming lessons. The next most frequently cited activities were bicycling and tricycling, taking walks, physical education classes, gymnastics and tumbling, roller skating, ice skating, dancing lessons, fun runs, school soccer, and downhill skiing.

Altogether, the parents in our study named fifty different sports and recreational activities in which their one- to thirteen-year-old children were involved. These activities accommodated a range of different interests, ages, and skills, and were available to children in several settings. If you are looking for ways to get your child involved, you might be interested to know some of the more common activities that cropped up in our survey:

1. Intra- and extramural sports programs and school physical education classes offer obvious opportunities for team or individual sports. Depending on their age, physical maturation, and mental readiness, children can get involved in swimming, soccer, volleyball, hockey, track and field, and a host of other sports.

2. Community recreation programs offer softball, T-ball, Little League, fun runs, tumbling and gymnastics, Jr. Jazzercise, and yoga.
3. Programs designed specifically for younger children include YMCA or YWCA infant exercise and parent–child exercise classes, swimming classes, or private programs such as Babygym, Kindergym, Tinytots, and gymboree.
4. Some children will enjoy group or private lessons in dance, tennis, skating, or other activities.
5. Summer camps, scouting clubs, and programs like Outward Bound provide a multitude of unique opportunities to combine physical activity fun with learning specific skills, self-reliance, getting along in the outdoors, and cooperation with others.
6. Children can engage in many of the activities mentioned so far on a more informal basis with their friends or family. Outings or trips can include bicycling, walks, hiking, backpacking, canoeing, cross-country skiing, jogging . . . the possibilities are endless!

Whatever activities your children choose, at some point of physical readiness and sufficient interest you should encourage them to participate in one or two aerobic "lifetime" activities. Cycling, swimming, hiking, or cross-country skiing are activities that won't end with graduation from high school or college; they can be enjoyed at any age. According to Dr. Roy Shepard of the University of Toronto, sports that keep children active for long periods of time are also more likely to keep them permanently involved in physical activity.

THE BENEFITS OF PHYSICAL ACTIVITY FOR CHILDREN

As with adults, regular physical activity provides a multitude of physical, psychological, and social benefits. William Strong, M.D., pediatrics professor and director of the Georgia Institute for the Prevention of Human Disease and Accidents, and Jack Wilmore, Ph.D., kinesiology professor at the University of Texas at Austin, have written about the many ways they believe children can benefit from regular physical activity, and ultimately, from physical fitness. Regular activity can improve children's appearance, control their weight, control mild hypertension, improve their posture, and improve overall functional and motor abilities. Psychologically, active children have a greater sense of well-being and lower anxiety levels.

These benefits and many other benefits of physical activity for children were confirmed by Melpomene's 1986 survey. Children, from toddlers to teenagers, who are more physically active, are more likely to have better overall physical health, coordination, motor development, strength, flexibility, and regular sleeping patterns. Active kids also tend to recuperate more quickly from illness. Regular physical activity, when performed with at least a moderate level of vigorousness, can begin to develop aerobic capacity for healthier heart and lungs, particularly for maturing adolescents.

The psychological benefits of participating in sports and recreational activities are equally important. Mastering an activity can give kids self-confidence, while enhancing their body image and their self-esteem. Their sense of accomplishment grows each time they take on and succeed in a new physical challenge. As they watch themselves improve, they begin to appreciate their bodies and trust their own physical potential. Once children get a sense of how good it feels to be fit, they will always have a built-in incentive to keep exercising, even into adulthood.

The social benefits of participating in physical activities are also numerous. Through informal, active games or organized sports, children learn to get along with others, work as part of a team, and handle losing or failure. When the entire family participates, the relationships between parents and children are usually enhanced. These social skills will serve children later in life, when the team atmosphere switches to the office, or when they are developing relationships with their own children.

TOO MUCH, TOO SOON? MINIMIZING NEGATIVE EXPERIENCES

So far, it would appear nothing critical can be said of physical activity for children. Overall, its benefits far outweigh any disadvantages or negative impacts. By keeping in mind a few basic considerations, parents, physicians, teachers, and coaches can minimize or avoid negative consequences and can help make sports and recreation positive experiences for children.

John Thatcher cautions parents to bear in mind that children's attention spans are shorter than adults', and that youngsters may not be enthusiastic about activities that require a great amount of time or concentration, like jogging or golf. Attempting to keep children involved in your favorite activity may not help promote their interests. Instead, we suggest you give your kids lots of options and allow them to quit certain activities and try new ones. Children will have more freedom to discover activities they enjoy, including ones that they might stick with for a lifetime.

Sometimes, in our eagerness to see our children embrace physical activity, we may inadvertently sour their experience. Parental or coaching pressures to start at too young an age, spend too much time, or train too intensively or competitively can turn off most children. When children's muscles and bones are still developing, they can be quite susceptible to pain and injuries if pushed too hard. Equally traumatic is the potential for emotional stress. Children will quickly sense if you have expectations about their performance or if you put a high value on competition. They can become easily frustrated and actually lose self-esteem and confidence if they don't feel they are living up to your expectations. They can also become disenchanted with a sport if they are too young to understand directions or team-play concepts, or if they are too emotionally or socially immature for the disciplined group interaction demanded by some sports. Pay close attention to your child's reactions; kids need encouragement to continue to achieve.

THE FUN ROAD TO FITNESS FOR CHILDREN

Children's natural inclination for physical activity can be further stimulated and guided by parents, schools, and community programs. By setting good examples and providing encouragement and opportunities, adults can open the doors to children for enjoyable, safe, and health-enhancing recreation and sports.

The following guidelines can make this endeavor easier and more successful. As a parent you can:

- Be active yourself. "Do as I say, *and* as I do!"
- Make time for physical activity and recreation as a family.

- Discuss your children's specific interests and let them choose activities they enjoy most.
- Show enthusiasm and support for their accomplishments without expecting superior athletic achievements.
- Invite them to walk or bike with you as an alternative to travel by car.
- Provide opportunities for taking lessons or classes, going to camp, or joining scouting clubs offering physical activities.
- Help your children set goals that are reasonable and achievable for their age, physical maturation, psychological readiness, and individual physical abilities.
- Talk to them about how they are feeling—physically and emotionally—to help avoid potential injuries or emotional anxieties stemming from sports participation.
- Include them on camping, hiking, canoeing, skiing, and other trips and outings.
- Encourage activities that do not involve excessive competition, training, or physical contact beyond your children's physical or psychological capabilities.
- Emphasize enjoyment and personal improvement over "win, win, win" or "no pain, no gain."
- Promote lifelong sports like swimming, cycling, tennis, jogging, skiing, or hiking.

Getting your children involved in sports and recreation is a great way to help them cultivate a lifelong exercise habit. The benefits are far-reaching, in terms of immediate and long-term gains in health and well-being. Help them discover that fitness is fun!

ENCOURAGING YOUR ACTIVE TEENAGER

The teenage years can be an emotional roller coaster. As we move from childhood to adulthood, it can feel like the whole world is watching us, and that our very worth depends on whether or not we are popular. Our peer group becomes the critical panel of experts, setting the bounds for what is acceptable, and more important, what is "cool."

Thankfully, sports for girls is becoming more acceptable all the time as our societal image of an attractive woman expands to include descriptors such as "toned," "in shape," and "healthy looking." The fact that more girls are involved in physical activity is encouraging, especially since the results of our 1983 membership survey show clearly that women who are involved in physical activity later in life commonly developed this interest at a young age. The teenage years are often a proving ground that determines whether a physically active adolescent will continue this passion into adulthood.

Encouragement can be an all-important factor in whether a girl follows her inclination to be active. Unfortunately, girls still do not get the same amount of encouragement in the sports arena as boys do. In a roundtable discussion with our staff, several teenage girls from the Twin Cities in Minnesota talked about the support they receive and how it differs from what boys receive.

Says Melanie, "I think that one of the reasons guys take sports much more seriously is because the people watching them do. People go to their games, and the next day they are talking about everything that happened and it's really a big deal. When we talk about our games, it's 'taking it too far.' " About personal support, she says, "My brother is in eighth grade this year. I have noticed how my dad treated us when we were both in sports. My dad would get a little more excited about what my brother was doing . . . My dad would support me, but he wouldn't get all gung ho about it and take a bunch of pictures like he did with my brother." Katy says, "Occasionally, I would come home and I would say, 'Dad, I swam my best time,' and then he would turn to Ken and ask him how his practice was. It was a little bit hard at first, but I know my dad wasn't doing it intentionally. I guess after four years with me and my sister [our accomplishments] got to be old hat."

Eva Auchincloss, cofounder and former executive director of the Women's Sports Foundation, addressed this issue in a panel discussion on the importance of girls' participation in sports. She first related a story of a high-school swimming team that had twenty nationally ranked swimmers and had beaten all its major rivals to place in the top of the nation.

Despite this achievement, said Auchincloss, the school hadn't given the girls one iota of recognition. "That same school, however, had praised the boys' football team in the assembly and awarded it honors, even though it had only one all-American and a mediocre win/loss record. The principal attended the boys' games and not once attended the girls' swim meets. The girls had to go up to the principal's office, tell him of their success and ask to have their picture taken with him so that they would have some memento of their accomplishments."

Is it any wonder that some girls are not as interested in sports as boys are? What can you as a parent or teacher do to encourage your teenage girls to be active? In one of our brochures on fitness for teenagers, Melpomene offers the following tips.

As adults we can:

- Exercise with teenagers.
- Talk about our own physical activity.
- Ask girls about their sport or team.
- Watch for compulsive exercising behavior that may be indicative of other behavior problems.
- Talk about sport and fitness opportunities outside of school and after graduation.
- Be supportive of the time commitment needed to practice or compete in sports.
- Encourage athletic directors to hire qualified women to coach girls' teams.
- Learn the details of your daughter's (or students') activity.
- Encourage girls to try a variety of activities—recreational as well as competitive.
- *Be a fan!*

There is good reason to play this role for your daughters or students. As we have mentioned, the physically active person has a much better chance of enjoying good health throughout his or her lifetime. Also, the psychological benefits of a play break can provide a kind of ongoing therapy for life. Sociability and the opportunity to form friendships is also something that sports can offer throughout life. One by-product that is often not talked about, however, is the important role sports play in the socialization process. As Eva Auchincloss states in her speech:

> Feeling the support of family, friends, school, and community is essential to developing the character of those who are going to become self-confident and able citizens. But play and sport [which is organized play] offer the arena in which the strongest socializing factors in any society are revealed. For it is through our play/sports that we act out the values that society wants us to assimilate; and it's in our games that we test our strength, ability, and fortitude. It is my belief that women and men who have had to test their will, determination, and ability through sports are more capable of self-determination later in life. I base this on my gut feeling and on the enormous amount of research that has been done [mostly on men] that correlates goal orientation, self-sufficiency, self-discipline, commitment, self-confidence, and assertiveness with "success' as it is defined by our society—leadership in one's field of endeavor.
>
> I believe that we learn the right stuff on the playing field and that the myth in our society is that girls are given the same encouragement and chance to participate on that playing field as boys. It is not only laws, money, and playing schedules that will make a difference, but you, the parents and grandparents who value and care as much about what your girls do as what your boys do.

S I X

AGE AND THE ACTIVE WOMAN

When people say we are "aging gracefully," they are usually referring to our physical appearance. But the real secret of aging well has nothing to do with looks; it's all attitude. One of our older members has a great comeback for women who say they are dreading the aging process. "If you're worried about getting old," she says, "just think of the alternative!"

Aging is part of moving forward in life, a process we all begin at birth. As women, we experience a second "coming of age" when we start to lose our hormones, signaling the end of our reproductive years and the beginning of menopause. This transition into a new stage of life is a time to consider our past struggles, our current abilities, and our future potential. In most developed countries of the world, women can expect to live thirty years or more after menopause. Women preparing for these years are inundated with articles and advertisements about special diets and exercise programs, all of which come with glowing "guarantees" for a healthier old age. Naturally, there is some confusion on the part of women who are trying to ferret out factual information about what they can do to enhance their later years.

You may have asked yourself some of these same questions: Will I have to slow down? Should I take calcium supplements? What about vitamin D? Phosphorus? Protein? Can I start biking, swimming, skating, or cross-country skiing at sixty? How will exercise affect my health? My attitude? My self-esteem? Will exercising regularly mean I'll look ten years younger? In this chapter, we'll explore some of these questions by looking at the changes you can expect in the second half of your life, the role that exercise can play in your new lifestyle, and ways to alleviate menopausal discomfort and lessen your risk of osteoporosis.

WHAT CAN WE EXPECT?

LIFESTYLE CHANGES

As our life span grows longer, the concept of aging takes on new meaning. Because life expectancies now stretch into the seventies and eighties, the "midlife" years creep into the fifties, and the sixties seem younger than they once did. At Melpomene, where we are privileged to work with very active senior volunteers and master athletes, we've learned to gauge a woman not by the number of years that she's been alive but by how alive she feels, acts, and looks today.

In addition to the physical changes we'll discuss next, we can all look forward to some type of lifestyle change in our later years. After several decades of working and/or raising a family, a whole new segment of life can open when the last child leaves or when retirement begins. If we have our health, there is no end to the new frontiers we can begin to explore. It can be a time for travel, for going back to school, or for realizing the dreams of a second career. It can also be a release from time pressures, when many women, perhaps for the first time, finally have time for themselves. For those of us who haven't ever made time for physical activity, the second half of life is an excellent time to start playing. There are many ways to combine travel and activity, such as walking tours, biking vacations, or other outdoor excursions. Grandchildren can be another wonderful entree to the world of play. They are built-in partners, and romping with them in the park or backyard can put us back in touch with our physical self.

Physical activity can also come in handy as a stress reducer in later years, when some of the changes we must face feel beyond our control. Consider, for instance, that most of us are likely to experience divorce, separation, or the death of a partner in our later years. Eleven out of twelve wives will become widows, and the average American woman can expect ten years of widowhood. The death of a partner is probably the greatest emotional upheaval, but divorce, which occurs in one-third of all first marriages, certainly comes close. If a divorce or separation occurs after many years of marriage, the change in a woman's role and status can be a frightening adjustment.

Feeling healthy and in touch with your body can be a bright spot on the horizon, helping you work your way back from these low and lonely times. Joining active groups can put you in contact with other people who share your interests. The social function of exercise cannot be overstated, especially when you consider that half of all women over forty years old live alone. The companionship of a walking partner or a tennis friend can be a lifeline, adding a dimension of hope and playfulness to any life.

PHYSICAL CHANGES

Following is a list of the normal changes that you may encounter with aging. Of course, you may not experience each and every one of these changes; aging varies with the individual and is affected by genetic and environmental factors. The timing of these changes is also difficult to pinpoint because it varies from person to person.

System	Changes
Integumentary (skin)	Lines and wrinkles
	Thinning and dryness
Musculoskeletal	Loss of flexibility of joints
	Loss of bone density
Endocrine	Decrease in hormones
	Decrease in basal metabolism
Sensory changes	Decreased sight
	Progressive hearing loss
	Loss of taste sensation
	Decreased sense of smell
	Decreased ability to distinguish hot or cold
Neurological	Slowing down of reaction time
	Changing sleep patterns
	Diminished short-term memory

System	Changes
Gastrointestinal	Slowing down of peristalsis
	Decreased ability to absorb and use minerals and nutrients
Genitourinary	Decreased muscle tone
	Decreased bladder capacity
	Thinning and drying of the vaginal walls
Cardiovascular	Increase in size of the heart
	Thickening of the valves and blood vessels
	Decrease in supply of blood to organs and extremities

Sometimes these normal changes of aging affect how we function in the world. They limit us in new ways, and we find ourselves wishing we could do the things we were once able to do. Do you find, for instance, that kneeling in the garden is not as easy or as comfortable as it once was? Do you have to make two or three lists just to keep track of what must be done in a day?

Are you staying indoors more days than you wish because of stress incontinence? These changes are not only frustrating but also wearing on your mental and emotional well-being. Our physical limitations can lead to isolation, stress, and feelings of depression, loss, or confusion. Masking the grief that is sometimes associated with aging can lead to alcoholism or other addictive behaviors.

The following story by Virginia tells us how depression around the time of her menopause was affecting her health:

> I was depressed for what seemed years around my menopause. I coped by "numbing out" with alcohol, resulting in my not being there for my kids. I felt unhealthy, fatigued, headachy, and out of shape. With help from friends and therapy, I first tackled my physical well-being; feeling better, with my self-esteem higher, I was then able to uncover the areas I really needed to work on in therapy. Eventually, I learned to manage my depression and opt for changes in my life.

Our health is obviously tied to our emotional as well as our physical state. By working on both, Virginia was able to make her way out of the depression that had held her hostage during her menopause. She began by making changes in her diet and her exercise regime that took into account the limits and possibilities of her changing, aging body. Accepting and becoming comfortable with her body's new "house rules" was the first step in restoring her lost vitality and self-esteem.

MENOPAUSE

Menopause is a developmental landmark for all women. It is a tangible transition that signals "aging has begun," and is medically defined as the day the last menstrual period ends. The menstrual flow stops because the body is no longer producing as much estrogen and progesterone as it once did. This change in hormone production is a normal part of the aging process. When there are no longer enough hormones to build up the lining of the uterus each month, the monthly flow stops and menopause begins. Menopause can also be brought on surgically by removing the ovaries and, usually, the uterus. These procedures are called bilateral oophorectomy and hysterectomy.

Not all healthcare providers see menopause in the same light. Some subscribe to a "disease model" of menopause based on the thinking that the menopausal woman is estrogen deficient. Menopause is seen as a departure from the "normal," or reproductive phase, of a woman's life. In this framework, menopause is a diagnosed condition, recognized by laboratory tests and doctor's examinations. R. A. Wilson, in his 1966 book *Feminine Forever*, made explicit the concept of menopause as disease and likened woman's future without estrogen to a sort of living decay, "in a negative state: dependent, vapid, unfortunate, unseeing, and without vigor."

Wilson's viewpoint is in direct contrast to looking at the menopause as a natural event in which the woman's self-knowledge and awareness of her body leads her to conclude that she is menopausal. In this framework, menopause is neither a disorder nor a departure from the norm. Rather, menopause is a perfectly healthy part of being a woman. As you might imagine, we subscribe to this school of thought. Below you'll find a list of the more common signs to help you recognize your own menopause, as well as some techniques that have helped other women.

SIGNS OF MENOPAUSE AND WAYS TO BE MORE COMFORTABLE

Menstrual Irregularity/Cessation of Menstruation. The period of change is gradual, often starting when a woman is in her mid- to late forties and lasting five to seven years. Periods may stop abruptly or become irregular or occasionally heavy before tapering off. Heavy bleeding is often the most annoying and worrisome symptom. You will find in talking with your friends or looking at your mother's history of menopause that each individual's experience is unique.

Vaginal Changes. As estrogen levels in your body diminish, your vagina may become shorter, narrower, and less elastic. The walls will lose their ability to lubricate, causing them to itch or burn especially during sex. Regular sexual activity, if not too uncomfortable, can keep the vaginal walls lubricating, even when they have become thinner. You can also lubricate and/or massage the walls of the vagina and vulva area yourself with the following balms:

> Vegetable oils: safflower, coconut, cocoa butter (don't use Vaseline, cold cream, or mineral oils—they can irritate the tissue or block secretions)
> Aloe Vera Gel
> Vitamin E capsules (puncture and use the oil)

Urinary Changes. The lining of the bladder and urethra may also become thin and dry, causing higher risk of bladder infections, incontinence, and having to urinate more often during the night. In some women the muscles in the bladder and urethra become weaker. This muscle weakening may lead to a loss of bladder control known as stress incontinence. For example, you may lose a little urine when you cough, sneeze, or laugh. Kegel exercises are a simple set of exercises that may help you strengthen the muscles that control urine flow.

Kegel exercises were devised some thirty years ago by Dr. Arnold

Kegel to help women with stress incontinence. They are designed to strengthen the pubococcygeus, the muscle that encircles the urethra (urinary opening) and the outside walls of the vagina. Many women find that these exercises also help increase sexual awareness while stimulating vaginal lubrication. This lubrication can help prevent the dryness that occurs with menopause.

Before you can do the exercises, you must first locate the pubococcygeus (P.C.) muscle. Sit on the toilet, spread your legs apart, and try to stop the flow of urine midstream without moving your legs. The P.C. muscle is the one you use to stop the urine. Now that you know where it is and what it feels like, you can begin the strengthening exercises.

First tighten the P.C. muscle as you did to stop the urine. Hold it for a count of three. Relax. Repeat the exercise ten times, several times a day. Build to twenty-five to thirty repetitions about five times a day. You can do the contractions anywhere and at any time throughout the day—while driving a car, sitting at a desk, watching TV, waiting for the elevator, or lying in bed. Remember to breathe naturally while doing your Kegels. If you practice these exercises frequently, you will notice improved muscle tone within a few weeks or a few months.

Hot Flashes. Nurse and researcher Ann Voda describes a hot flash as a sudden sensation of heat or a warm feeling as perceived and determined through the self-report of women. Other sensations include tingling, throbbing, a "rush of blood," light-headedness, chills, and the feeling of suffocation. While most women can expect some form of hot flashes during menopause, the frequency and the length of years you experience them may vary widely from woman to woman. The "triggers" for hot flashes also vary among women. The common denominator is that hot flashes can be very uncomfortable. Below is a list of suggestions that may help alleviate some of the discomfort:

Eat slowly and avoid hot liquids and spicy foods.
Drink ice water and use cold compresses on your face.
Take a cool bath and splash cool water on your face.
Cool yourself with a fan.
Dress in layers so you can peel some off.

Dissolve 1 cup table salt in a bathtub of warm water and lie in the
   tub until the water cools.
Work at eliminating stress; use relaxation techniques.

Other related signs of menopause are headaches, swollen ankles, insomnia, skin tingling, numbness, fatigue, depression, irritability, and
anxiety.

It's important to be good to yourself when your body is undergoing
so many changes. A diet that is high in fresh vegetables, fruit, beans, and
whole grains, and low in red meats and saturated fats, may bring relief
from many of these symptoms. Exercising during this time will not only
boost your mental well-being but will also strengthen and tone your muscles, improve your circulation, digestion, and elimination, and help you
prevent osteoporosis.

HORMONE REPLACEMENT THERAPY

Since menopause is characterized by a decrease in estrogen, doctors began
to experiment with estrogen supplements in the 1960s. Estrogen replacement therapy became touted as a veritable fountain of youth, promising
to help women prevent wrinkles, maintain a youthful silhouette, and keep
their hair luxuriant and shiny while eliminating hot flashes, depression,
and uncomfortable sexual activity (due to drying and thinning of the
vaginal walls). The balloon burst in the late 1970s when researchers found
that estrogen users were six to fourteen times more likely to develop endometrial (uterine) cancer than nonusers. Since then, estrogen doses have
been lowered and progesterone has been added in hopes of imitating more
closely the balance of hormones in a natural menstrual cycle. This combination is thought to prevent the building up of the endometrium (the
lining of the uterus) to a precancerous state. However, results from a 1989
study conducted by Dr. Bergkvist and colleagues at the University Hospital in Uppsala, Sweden, have shown the possibility of an increase in
risk of breast cancer among women receiving hormone replacement therapy, especially among those women who were taking progesterone. While
the results of this study are by no means conclusive, they do point to a
need for reevaluation and further study of the risks associated with hormone replacement therapy.

The influence of estrogen goes beyond the menstrual cycle. Researchers have shown, for instance, that estrogen is the single most important variable in the prevention of bone loss in postmenopausal women. For this reason, estrogen is sometimes prescribed as way to prevent osteoporosis, or thinning of the bones. According to Bruce Ettinger, M.D., University of California Medical Center at San Francisco, the longer a woman takes estrogen, the more skeletal benefits she derives. Because it is difficult to measure bone loss directly, researchers can only gauge whether or not estrogen is working by tracking how many bone fractures occur. Ettinger now feels that there is ample evidence showing that estrogen reduces the risk of fracture by half.

In many hospitals and clinics, the use of estrogen supplements has become almost automatic. Some physicians are likely to prescribe estrogen for menopausal women without even asking the woman how she feels about it.

> *It is just routine here; when a woman comes in and complains of hot flashes, she is prescribed estrogen. Menopause means estrogen . . . period.*
> —NURSE PRACTITIONER, MIDWEST OB-GYN CLINIC

You should be aware that there is a wide range of opinion among physicians regarding estrogen replacement. Some feel it is a cure-all and others are hesitant to prescribe it. The following list describes the risks and benefits of taking estrogen. If you are considering the use of hormones, read this list and write down all your questions and concerns before you go to your doctor. Ask your physician to explain what you personally could expect to gain and what you might risk by taking hormones. Make sure all of your questions have been answered before you make your decision.

BENEFITS

Reduces risk of osteoporosis
Eliminates hot flashes, depression, and other symptoms associated with menopause
Reduces vaginal dryness
Possibly reduces risk of heart attack

RISKS

Increased risk of gallbladder disease
Possible return of periods and/or cramping
Nausea and vomiting
Swelling of the ankles, feet, and fingers
Bloating
Breast tenderness

REASONS WHY YOU MAY NOT BE ABLE TO TAKE ESTROGEN

History of uterine or breast cancer
History of thrombotic disorders (formation of blood clots)
Diabetes
Hypertension
Unexplained vaginal bleeding
History of gallbladder or liver disease

Hormone replacement is not necessarily for everyone. You need to discuss your specific expectations and needs with your physician, and carefully weigh the possible risks you may face. If you decide that you would benefit from hormone replacement, you will want to closely monitor your health while you receive it. Your yearly physical examinations should include a breast examination and possibly a mammogram, a Pap smear, and a blood pressure reading.

As we mentioned above, estrogen is now given in lower dosages and is combined with progesterone. There are several regimes given, some that are accompanied by bleeding and some that are not. To be effective, estrogen should be combined with a high calcium intake (1,500 mg/day) and regular exercise.

OSTEOPOROSIS

Fact: One out of every four postmenopausal women has osteoporosis.
Fact: Osteoporosis accounts for one million hip, wrist, and spine
   fractures annually in U.S. citizens over age forty-five.
Fact: Women are eight times more likely than men to develop osteoporosis.

Osteoporosis, symbolized by the dowager's hump, feared for its brittle
bones, and characterized by its insidious, silent progression, is a major
health problem in the United States. From *osteo* meaning bones, and
porosis meaning full of holes, this age-related disorder is characterized by
decreased bone mass with increased susceptibility to fractures.

To understand how we lose bone mass, it helps to know something
about bone building and remodeling that goes on in our bodies. Our
bones are not static—they are constantly breaking down and rebuilding,
usually in a balance that keeps them strong. Estrogen, calcium, and exercise play major roles in this remodeling process. Weight-bearing exercise and calcium help to build bone mass, while estrogen slows the process
of bone breakdown. When any of these elements are in low supply, breakdown can start to outpace buildup, leading to weakened, porous bones,
a condition known as osteoporosis.

When bones are thin and full of holes, they become brittle. A minor
fall or something as simple as bending over to make a bed can cause a
woman with osteoporosis to break a bone or compress her spinal verte-
brae. According to Steven R. Cummings, M.D., about 247,000 hip
fractures occurred in persons over age forty-five in 1986. In people over
sixty-five, this incidence of hip fracture rises dramatically; by age eighty,
a Caucasian woman runs a 1 percent to 2 percent annual risk of suffering
a hip fracture. About 15 percent of Caucasian women suffer a hip fracture at some point in their lives. Fractures of the wrist, commonly called
Colles' fracture, are another common consequence of osteoporosis. A fifty-
year-old Caucasian woman runs about a 15 percent risk of breaking her
wrist because of her porous bones. Men and blacks are not as likely to
suffer from osteoporosis as Caucasian women.

Besides bone breakage, the most common structural change associated with osteoporosis is the dowager's hump, a permanent spinal deformity that can cause a woman to lose at least 15 percent of her height. Therefore, a woman who has been 5'4" could lose up to nine inches by the time she reaches eighty. About 40 percent of all women will have at least one wedge-type spinal deformity by the time they reach eighty. One woman writes:

> Two years ago my mother who is eighty-two fractured her hip after a fall. The physicians weren't sure if she fell and broke her hip or if the hip gave way first. They said she has osteoporosis. I always thought women become "stooped over" because of the burdens they'd carried for years . . . I've just turned sixty, and I noticed that I've lost over an inch in height . . . What is my risk for a hip fracture? Will I have osteoporosis since my mother has been diagnosed with it?

WHO IS AT RISK FOR OSTEOPOROSIS?

As women watch their mothers growing shorter each year, they wonder whether they themselves are at risk for osteoporosis. As you can see from the list below, there are definite risk factors that are not under our control: family history, ancestry, being female, and premature menopause. Other factors that put us at risk for osteoporosis are under our control. These factors mainly include lifestyle habits: level of physical activity, calcium intake, cigarette smoking, and alcohol and caffeine use.

THE RISK FACTORS OF OSTEOPOROSIS

1. Premature menopause (natural or surgical)
2. Nulliparity (no history of childbirth)
3. Family history of osteoporosis
4. Northern European ancestry
5. Slender body build, fair skin, blond or reddish hair
6. Being female
7. Associated medical conditions that can independently result in accelerated bone loss, for example, gastrectomy, anorexia, diabetes, kidney or liver disease

Other risk factors that are under a person's control are:

1. Low level of physical activity
2. Low level of calcium intake
3. Lifestyle habits: smoking, caffeine, and alcohol use
4. Inadequate fluoride level in the water supply
5. Being confined indoors
6. Ingestion of drugs: anticonvulsants, corticosteroids, antacids containing aluminum (inhibit absorption of calcium) and diuretics (increase the excretion of calcium)

HOW IS OSTEOPOROSIS DETECTED?

The symptoms of osteoporosis are fractures, the dowager's hump, and the loss of height. There are no laboratory tests that will tell you whether you are at risk or whether you already have mild osteoporosis. Ordinary x-rays don't detect osteoporosis clearly until 30 percent of bone mineralization is already lost. There are techniques that can measure smaller amounts of bone loss, but they are best used if you are in the high-risk category, or if you are facing a decision about estrogen use. The costs of the procedures are listed below:

Technique	Cost	Sites Measured
Single-photon	$40–120	Hand and wrist
Dual-photon	$150–300	Spine and hip
CT scan	$100–300	Spine

Radiation exposure is relatively low in these scanning techniques, but since radiation poses cancer risks, many women are hesitant to have scans unless they are really necessary. We agree that routine screening for osteoporosis is simply not justified. You'll probably do more for your health by understanding the risk factors and incorporating preventive measures into your lifestyle.

If you do find yourself at risk for osteoporosis, or if your bone mass is already weakened, what treatment options are available to you? Calcium, of course, has been shown to be important in maintaining bone mass, as have estrogen and exercise. We'll discuss the various options below.

CALCIUM AND OSTEOPOROSIS

In 1984, speakers at the National Institute of Health Conference on Osteoporosis recommended that American women should significantly increase the amount of calcium in their diets. While some researchers charged that these recommendations were premature, the message was clearly out. Since then, hundreds of articles in newspapers and magazines and dozens of television talk shows have focused on osteoporosis and on the role of calcium in preventing brittle bones. As soon as osteoporosis became a household word, marketing departments across the country got busy. Suddenly, a variety of foods from orange juice to cereal were being fortified with calcium. Advertisers played up the calcium content of familiar products such as Tums, which is now perhaps better known as a calcium supplement than as an antacid.

The media focus on calcium is somewhat misleading, however, because calcium alone will not prevent osteoporosis. Estrogen and exercise are also key players in this complex condition. Yet, a high-calcium intake may be beneficial for what is called age-related bone loss. Age-related bone loss occurs ten to fifteen years after menopause, and therefore is not related to estrogen deficiency. Researchers believe that this bone loss occurs, in part, because the gastrointestinal tract becomes less efficient at absorbing calcium as we get older. This problem is often compounded when women do not take in enough calcium. Studies have shown that an adequate calcium intake can reduce the rate of this age-related bone loss in the elderly.

Increasing calcium through diet or by taking supplements is only part of the story, however. Other factors in your diet or your lifestyle may actually be blocking calcium absorption or causing you to excrete it quickly. A good nutritional program of prevention, therefore, stresses (1) calcium intake, either in natural form, from supplements, or from a combination of the two, and (2) avoiding factors that adversely affect calcium absorption or excretion. See the table below for a list of what influences calcium absorption and excretion.

FACTORS THAT INFLUENCE CALCIUM ABSORPTION

Vitamin D. Vitamin D increases calcium absorption from the intestine and reabsorption from the kidneys. The recommended amount is 400 mg/day. Note, however, that an excess of this vitamin is not only toxic but also causes bone loss.

Fluoride. Fluoridated water promotes calcium retention and bone formation.

Protein. Red meat is high in phosphorus, a nutrient that prevents calcium absorption. Too much protein, however, can increase calcium excretion.

Sodium. The more sodium we eat, the more calcium we excrete.

Caffeine and alcohol. They act as diuretics and increase the loss of calcium through the urine. Alcohol also interferes with calcium absorption.

Phyates. Foods containing phyates may also make calcium unavailable for absorption, for example, oatmeal and bran.

Oxalates. Foods containing oxalic acid in combination with calcium interfere with absorption. Examples are spinach, rhubarb, sorrel, parsley, and beet greens. Vary these foods in your diet and do not use them as a main source of calcium.

Fiber. It interferes with absorption by combining with calcium in the intestine and by increasing the rate at which food is passed through the intestinal tract.

You don't have to eliminate any of these foods from your diet. In fact, fiber is essential and should not be eliminated. Oat bran is also helpful in reducing cholesterol levels in your blood. If your calcium intake is borderline, these foods should not be eaten at the same meal as the food you depend on for calcium.

What Is the RDA for Calcium? Dr. Robert Heaney, from Creighton University, recommends a daily calcium intake of between 1,000 and 1,500 mg/day. This is a significant increase from the former RDA of 800 mg, which was based on younger people's needs. The question is not only how much calcium you need but also how your body is using it. Some studies have shown that women should be consuming between 1,000 and 1,500 mg of calcium daily to prevent bone loss. Are you getting enough in your diet? Read the list below. Using the food journal on page 175, make a list of your daily intake of food and beverages, both in meals and snacks. Chances are that you are not consuming enough calcium in your diet. In our study, we found that only 24 percent of the total participants consumed more than 1,000 mg of calcium daily. In order to reach the recommended intake, the women would have had to either eat more calcium-rich foods or take calcium supplements.

CALCIUM SOURCES: ARE YOU GETTING ENOUGH BONE BUILDERS?

Milk (2%)—1 cup (300 mg)
Semisoft cheese—1 oz (200 mg)
Hard cheese—1 oz (300 mg)
Creamed cottage cheese—1 cup (150 mg)
Yogurt (plain)—1 cup (300 mg)
Grated Parmesan cheese—2 tablespoons (150 mg)
Vanilla ice cream—1 cup (170 mg)
Frozen yogurt—1 cup (200 mg)
Pudding—$\frac{1}{2}$ cup (150 mg)
Cheese sauce—$\frac{1}{2}$ cup (200 mg)
Cream of tomato soup—1$\frac{3}{4}$ cup (300 mg)
Pizza—2 slices (350 mg)
Hot cereal—1 cup (100 mg)
Pancakes—3 (milk added) (150 mg)
Custard pie—1 slice (150 mg)
Almonds—$\frac{1}{3}$ cup (100 mg)
Broccoli—1 cup (150 mg)
Greens (kale, Swiss chard, collard)—1 cup (300 mg)
Red salmon (canned with bones and oil)—4 oz (250 mg)
Sardines (canned with bones and oil)—2$\frac{1}{4}$ oz (350 mg)
Shrimp—4 oz (150 mg)

While calcium in food is probably more readily absorbed (thus making it the best choice), some women will find it difficult to consume the recommended amount. Melpomene finds that many women decide to use

FOOD JOURNAL

Food	Serving Size	Amount of Calcium
Breakfast		
Lunch		
Dinner		
Snacks		
Totals		

supplements to make up the difference. The next dilemma is choosing which kind of calcium supplement to take.

Calcium comes in three basic forms, each of which contains different amounts of usable calcium:

Type of Supplement	Amount of Usable (Elemental) Ca
Calcium carbonate	40 percent
Calcium lactate	13 percent
Calcium gluconate	9–10 percent

Since calcium carbonate has only 40 percent usable calcium, you'd only get 40 mg of calcium from a 100-mg tablet. Calcium gluconate gives you even less; you'd have to quadruple the dosage to wind up with the same amount of calcium you'd get if you took calcium carbonate.

To make sure you are getting what you need, look for one of two things:

1. The percentage of the U.S. RDA, for example, Each tablet contains 25 percent of USRDA calcium, 250 mg, or
2. The amount of usable or elemental calcium, that is, "Each tablet contains 500 mg of calcium carbonate, which provides 200 mg elemental (usable) calcium."

At Melpomene, we recommend that women take calcium carbonate, which not only provides the most usable calcium but is also generally the least expensive. We also caution women to avoid dolomite and bone meal, which are often contaminated by heavy metals such as lead.

Although supplements can be a good way to make sure you've gotten your calcium for the day, they are not without their problems. A few of the more common complaints about supplements include:

1. Large pill size. The pills are large because calcium is a bulky mineral. Alternatives include taking more pills of a smaller dosage, or using chewable tablets or powdered formulas. Be sure to space them out over the day and take with meals in order to enhance absorption. (See the warning above about foods that block absorption.)

2. High doses may cause constipation or gas. You might be able to avoid these problems by increasing your intake slowly over a couple of weeks. If you are still affected, try switching to another brand of supplement.
3. Kidney stones. There is no evidence that calcium alone will cause the formation of kidney stones. Most people can tolerate up to 2,000 mg/day without adverse effects. However, if you have a family history of kidney stones, or a predisposition to their formation, consult with your physician before you start taking supplements.

Besides dietary calcium and supplements, there are other factors that enhance bone building, including estrogen and exercise. In our experience, a three-pronged program of estrogen therapy, exercise, and calcium seems to offer the best protection against osteoporosis.

OSTEOPOROSIS AND EXERCISE

In 1982, Melpomene Institute began an ongoing osteoporosis study to answer questions about the relationship between long-term physical activity and bone density. The study group includes 111 female subjects, ages forty-nine to eight-three. Fifty-four of the subjects are classified as physically active and the other fifty-seven are in the physically inactive group. The participants in these two groups have been further sorted into six activity levels, based on exercise frequency, intensity, and duration.

Study participants were categorized into 6 groups,
each group reflecting an activity level of defined
intensity, frequency, and duration.

Low-Activity Group

Level 1. Sedentary
Very low daily household activity
Occasional flights of stairs, usually fewer than 2–3/day
Walks generally less than four blocks/day
No activity leading to a sweat

Level 2. Very Low Activity Level

Activity consists mainly of everyday living requirements—a few flights of stairs, a few blocks of walking, a relatively low level of housework

Usually no activity leading to a sweat

Medium-Activity Group

Level 3. Low Active

Activity revolves around maintaining household and family

No steady formal activity, however, she occasionally enjoys activities such as bowling, a bike ride, a walk, maybe some golf

Participation at any given time would be of short duration—less than one-half to one hour

Level 4. Moderately Active

Usually engages in very little "formal" athletic activity but leads a life that keeps her "on the go"

Frequent walks, several flights of stairs

Actively incorporates activity into her lifestyle as a complement to every-day activities

Activity is aerobic but at a low cardiovascular stress level

Length of any given activity would be one-half to one hour

High-Activity Group

Level 5. Very Active

Participates regularly, several times a week, in athletic activities

Actively incorporates activity into her lifestyle as a complement to every-day activities

Most compete at some level in one or more activities

Engages in activity for an hour 3–5 times per week

Level 6. Intensely Active

Participates in anaerobic activity at a high level (probably 70 percent of maximum heart rate) for an hour or more at a time, 5–7 days per week

High level of activity is as much a part of everyday living as all other aspects of life

Almost all compete in an activity

Source: Melpomene Report, Vol. 4, winter 1985.

Each of the women in our study completed a twelve-page questionnaire that included general health history, menstrual history, menopausal history, physical activity patterns, and lifestyle patterns. One hundred and seven subjects completed a three-day diet log that was analyzed with a computerized nutritional program. One hundred women underwent computerized tomography (CT) scans of the lumbar spine.

Our goal in this study was to provide factual information that would encourage women to incorporate good nutrition and exercise into their lifestyle. The underlying hypothesis was that women who have engaged in physical activity throughout their lives will have significantly denser bones (more bone mass) than their peers who did not engage in physical activity.

Indeed, this belief turned out to be true. The average bone density of the physically active women was 25.6 percent higher than the average of the women in the low-activity groups. Many studies besides our own confirm the finding that exercise does increase bone density and/or decrease significant bone loss in the postmenopausal woman.

How does exercise build bones? Everett L. Smith, Ph.D., explains that the two primary mechanical forces applied to bone are muscular contraction and the pull of gravity. Both are responsible for bone rebuilding. If either of these two forces is eliminated, bone mineral content starts to drop. For example, if you are on bedrest, without any weight-bearing or contraction-type exercise, your muscles will atrophy and your bones will lose density. Bone loss can also occur if you are only getting one type of exercise. For instance, in household chores like gardening and housework, the forces of muscle contraction are applied to the bone, but without a weight-bearing component. The resulting bone loss can be very significant if you are beyond the bone-building age of the mid-thirties or if you are menopausal. Women lose bone density at a rate of 0.75 to 1 percent each year beginning in their early thirties. During the five to ten years after menopause, this rate jumps to between 2 and 5 percent loss each year. The results in figures 6.2 and 6.3 will give you a feel for how bone density declined with the age of our subjects.

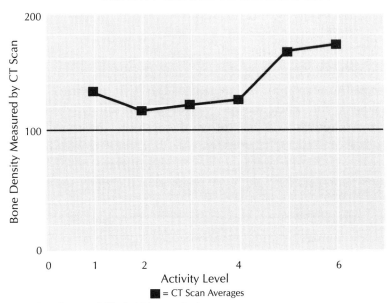

ACTIVITY RELATED TO BONE DENSITY

Source: New data compiled by the Melpomene Institute.

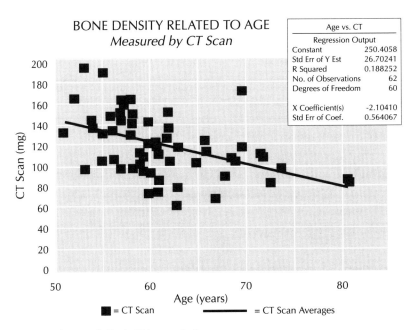

BONE DENSITY RELATED TO AGE
Measured by CT Scan

Age vs. CT	
Regression Output	
Constant	250.4058
Std Err of Y Est	26.70241
R Squared	0.188252
No. of Observations	62
Degrees of Freedom	60
X Coefficient(s)	-2.10410
Std Err of Coef.	0.564067

Source: New data compiled by the Melpomene Institute.

180

EXERCISES FOR THE PREVENTION AND MANAGEMENT OF OSTEOPOROSIS*

Women with osteoporosis are most likely to fracture a bone in the following areas: the upper arm at the shoulder, the forearm at the wrist, and the thighbone at the hip and spine. Only the hip and spine can be strengthened by weight-bearing exercises such as walking or running; the arms must be stressed with other specific exercises. The guidelines below will help you target the areas that need strengthening. Correct posture is also highlighted because it too can prevent certain types of fractures in porous bones.

Posture Correction. Sit straight and stand tall. Align your head directly over your spine. Trunk and limbs should be aligned over your base of support, which is your feet and the space in between. If you lean too far away from your base, you will become unstable and muscles may become strained. Maintain the natural curve of your low back at all times. Do not lock your knees.

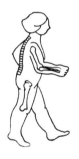

Posture Improvement: Standing and Sitting. Stand tall, with hands behind head. Pinch your shoulder blades together and press palms against the back of your head. Resist the forward movement by contracting your neck muscles also. Slowly contract and hold for five seconds, while breathing normally. Release slowly. Besides improving rounded shoulders and back, these exercises may also be used to avoid or lessen pain from existing osteoporotic spinal fractures. Sitting or lying

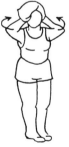
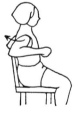

*Pages 181 to 185 by Diane E. Brodigan are reprinted with permission from *Melpomene Journal*.

positions are better in this case. When sitting, try slowly to press elbows toward the
back. Sit up straight and hold position for
five seconds.

Back Lying. With your arms perpendic-
ular to your trunk, bend elbows to ninety
degrees and press them into the floor.
Hold for five seconds, then relax.

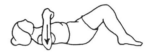

SPECIFIC EXERCISES FOR THE HIP AND SPINE SHOULD BE

1. Upright (standing).
2. Weight-bearing.
3. Endurance (aerobic), such as walking or mild jogging.
4. Performed for thirty minutes, three or four times per week.
5. Muscle strengthening, such as isometric abdominal contraction and
   back extension.

Endurance Activity. Begin continuous
walking with ten minutes a day. Gradually increase to thirty minutes a day. Always warm up first and use static stretch
before and after activity. Be sure to wear
cushioned, low-heeled walking or jogging
shoes. Legs, hip, and spine benefit from
working against gravity.

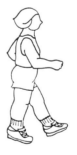

Isometric Abdominal Contraction. Lie on
back and press lower back against floor
and bend knees to ninety degrees. Tuck
chin to chest and contract abdominal
muscles. Hold position (while breathing
normally) for ten seconds. If osteoporosis
is present, avoid rolling shoulders off the
floor; attempt to keep the spine straight

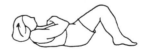

and pressed into the floor. Strong abdominal muscles protect the back against
strain. Remember: *Do not hold your
breath.*

Back Extension. Begin on all fours. With
back flat, lift one leg so that heel is level
with the buttocks, but no higher. Contract buttocks and thigh, and hold position for ten seconds. When your balance
improves, lift opposite arm simultane-
ously with the straight leg. Strengthens
the back, buttocks and hamstring (back
of the thigh).

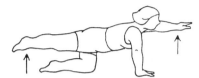

Specific Exercises for the Upper Body:
  1. Weight-loading: tension, torsion, compression, bending.
  2. Resistance exercise with a resistance stretch band: improves rounded
     shoulders and back by strengthening supporting muscles.

  Resistance stretch bands, such as Thera-Band, often can be purchased
from the rehabilitation/physical therapy department at your hospital. You
will need about one yard in length. The red band is low resistance; the
black is the highest resistance.

Tensile Loading. Hang from a bar or pull
on a doorknob for ten seconds. Avoid this
exercise if you have a wrist, elbow, or
shoulder injury.

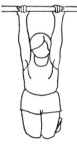

Torsion Loading. With a partner, bend elbows and grasp each other's wrists in position shown. Attempt to twist your arms in opposite directions against her resistance. Or, grasp a doorknob and twist wrist. Hold at maximum resistance for five seconds. Reverse direction.

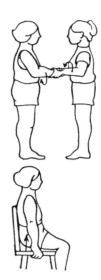

Compressive Loading: Sitting Push-ups. With feet on floor, grasp edge of chair seat. Straighten elbows (but do not lock them) to raise yourself one-half inch off the chair. Hold your weight on your hands for ten seconds, while breathing normally. Slowly bend elbows to lower yourself. Try hands in different positions: fingers pointing down, front or back. Bones become stronger and more dense when they must support weight and work muscles. *Avoid straining or holding your breath.* This may be difficult to do.

Compressive Loading/Bending. Begin on hands and knees with back flat. Contract abdominal muscles and buttocks to avoid a sagging back. Slowly bend your elbows to ninety degrees (if you can). Let your neck be a natural extension of your spine; do not hang your head. Push up by straightening your elbows. Try one arm alone, and use your fingertips. Or, place hands in different supporting positions: with arms crossed, with hands wider apart than shoulders, or "creep" hands forward and back while bending elbows. Try to keep your nose beyond an imaginary line between your fingertips.

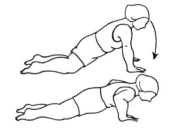

Resistance/External Rotation. Grasping Thera-Band, keep elbows pressed against your waist and slowly open forearms outward. Benefits shoulders and rounded back.

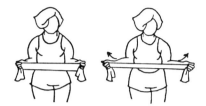

Resistance/Horizontal Abduction. Grasping Thera-Band, begin with arms straight in front, about chest height. Slowly open arms to the side. Do not lock your elbows or fling arms apart. Improves rounded shoulders and back.

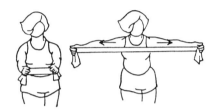

Positions to Avoid. Avoid slumping or forward bending of the spine when osteoporosis is present.

SOME FINAL THOUGHTS ON BONE LOSS

Even though the prevention of bone loss is a major concern of aging women, it should not be the only motivating force for exercise. Exercise and fitness have many benefits at all ages. Besides denser bones, exercise offers a sense of accomplishment, well-being, camaraderie, and a feeling of joy. Physically, exercise offers:

Increased work capacity; more energy
Lower resting and exercising heart rates
Lower blood pressure
Stronger, better-toned muscles
Flexible joints and ligaments

Older adults gain all the same benefits of exercise as younger people, but the experience of starting and sticking with a program can often be different. From our work with both active and inactive older women, we offer you the following food for thought.

EXERCISE AND THE OLDER WOMAN

". . . to be active in life is to be physically involved with life . . . since retirement, I've had more time to be physically active . . . I am more aware of the benefits of exercise."

"I started running when I was fifty-four. I quit smoking after thirty years, I'm now sixty and running is easier now than it has ever been. Exercise has increased my energy level and gives me a sense of well-being."

"I notice a restless feeling after a couple of days of no exercise."
—Participants, Melpomene Osteoporosis study

SHOULD OLDER WOMEN EXERCISE?

"I am a fifty-year-old woman who has been running for fitness and pleasure for the past seven years. Approaching menopause as I am, I am beginning to be concerned about various health issues. I find that the medical community has no experience with women who are as active as I am at my age. My healthcare provider thinks I shouldn't be running at all. I can't believe that it is all that bad, so I keep on."

A lot of menopausal women come to us with these same concerns. At this point, there is no conclusive evidence to prove that moderate exercise extends the lifespan of older adults. On the other hand, in the absence of major illness, no evidence of harm exists either. Rather, we can honestly say that a regular exercise regime can only improve an older adult's quality of life.

Results from our body image survey suggest that women who are physically active tend to have a more positive perception of "self" than women who are physically inactive. Though the self-perceptions of lower-activity women were not high on the scale, they did report that they were "satisfied" with their appearance and with their lower-energy and activ-

CURRENT HEALTH STATUS

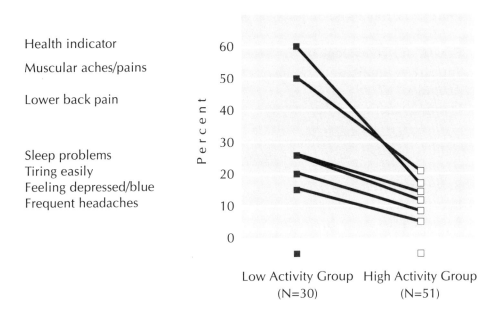

Health indicator

Muscular aches/pains

Lower back pain

Sleep problems
Tiring easily
Feeling depressed/blue
Frequent headaches

Low Activity Group   High Activity Group
(N=30)   (N=51)

ity levels. This finding is not surprising when you consider what we have traditionally deemed appropriate behavior for postmenopausal women. It concerned us, however, that the inactive women were not in good physical shape compared to the active group of women. The sedentary women reported more sleep problems, less energy, and more muscular aches and pains than the physically active women (above). Even though most of these women claimed to be "satisfied with themselves, 20 percent to 40 percent did express desire for change.

FACTORS THAT INFLUENCE EXERCISE

We wanted to know more than just how often and how intensely post-menopausal women exercise. We wanted to know why they did it, or why they didn't. The motivating or inhibiting factors that kept arising in our results included:

MOTIVATORS

Previous participation in physical education classes in secondary school
  and college
Education: knowledge of the benefits of activity
Support of family and friends
Attitudes
Personal health and fitness

INHIBITORS

Being overweight
Being a cigarette smoker
Being too far away from exercise facilities
Having too little time to participate

"Positive factors affecting my activity? The support and encouragement of my adult children, the availability of facilities, owning a
stationary bike for winter and foul weather, the incentive of upcoming runs or cross-country ski races, and personal goals. Bad weather
and 'other interests' keep me from my workouts at times."
—Connie, age fifty-five

"To maintain motivation for my exercise routine, I've found a partner . . ."
—Helga, age sixty-eight

Essential to motivation are the feelings of success and reward. All the
positive factors may be in place, but unless you have the motivation to
get up and get out there time and again, your success will be short-lived.
Rewards are excellent reinforcers of behavior. An example of a reward
might be going out to breakfast with your exercise partner or getting
yourself new walking shoes.
  Exercise should above all be fun: a chance to socialize, wear comfortable clothes and shoes, and do something physical for a change. Don't
overdo; walk with purpose, through a park, or to your favorite neighbor's

garden. Exercise is more likely to be enjoyable if it is not overly taxing or intense.

If you are an older woman who is just becoming physically active, you may be a pioneer in your community. All of us need to show, by our example, that exercise is both appropriate and healthful for older women. Of course, we need to paint a realistic picture as well, and be truthful with women who are just starting to become active. Some of the problems that may challenge these women are:

1. Lack of support of family and friends
   "My friends and relatives warned that I'll ruin my joints and my bladder will sag from all this running. This puzzles me because I feel so much better when I run."
2. Being regarded as old and infantile
   "My family may not want to believe it, but I *can* make my own decisions. I know what is good for me."
3. Having to alter or modify exercise patterns due to the normal aging process
   "Arthritis finally got the best of my daily walking routine. I miss the time with my friends but we get together for coffee or tea at the "Y" where I've taken up swimming . . . much easier on my hips and I still feel active and healthy."

These areas are difficult to confront. Often, as with other parts of the normal aging process, you have no control over the events that limit your abilities to maintain exercise patterns. Your ability to accept the changes and make modifications (without losing your enthusiasm) will make all the difference.

SOME TIPS FOR ENJOYABLE WORKOUTS

Whether you exercise on your own, with a partner, or with a group led by a leader, the warm-up and cool-down are important components in a safe and positive exercise experience. You can warm up by stretching or by doing the activity itself at a low intensity for the first few minutes.

The cool-down period after your workout brings the cardiovascular system to a recovery state slowly, and helps prevent soreness. Cool-down may include a slow walk, a low-intensity version of the activity, or a series of stretches.

The clothing you exercise in should be loose for freedom of movement (an oversized T-shirt), yet supportive where needed (e.g., athletic bras and cushioned socks). Shoes should also be well-cushioned and offer good arch and heel support with a nonskid sole.

Older adults need to use caution when exercising in hot conditions to avoid the dangers of rapid dehydration and heat stroke. Dehydration can be avoided by routinely drinking eight glasses of water per day, and then drinking plenty of water during and after exercise to replace lost fluids. Generally, if you follow this schedule of water replacement, the commercial electrolyte replacements will not be necessary.

Older adults should also use caution when exercising in the cold because of their tendency toward vasoconstriction—meaning the small vessels constrict, making the heart work harder to maintain the body's heat. Exposed areas such as the fingers, toes, ears, and head must be covered to prevent frostbite. Cover your head to prevent losing heat. The ideal activities in cold weather are those that cause you to generate your own body heat.

There are also other cautions you should know about when exercising. Below is a list of some warning signs that should tell you to stop exercising. Consult your physician or fitness instructor before resuming your exercise activities.

REASONS TO STOP EXERCISING

Dizziness
Chest pain
Shortness of breath or difficulty catching your breath
Nausea
Staggering or persistent unsteadiness
Mental confusion
Pallor around the lips
Profuse sweating along with heart palpitations
Sharp headache

What are good forms of exercise? Walking, jogging, cross-country skiing, tennis, bicycling, dancing, bowling, low-impact aerobics, calisthenics, and weight lifting are all good types of exercise for the older woman. You can maintain a reasonable level of fitness by engaging in an aerobic activity for at least thirty minutes three to four times per week. Even though swimming is not weight-bearing, it is considered a good form of exercise for the older woman. Because it puts almost no stress on the body, swimming is a great workout for someone who is arthritic or who has developed osteoporosis.

Walking is another all-round good physical activity that puts very little stress on the body. Walking, however, is weight-bearing, and thus helps to lessen the loss of bone mass that leads to osteoporosis. If you are interested in walking, try following the advice from our walking program instructors:

1. Start with ten minutes of easy walking at least three times a week.
2. Gradually walk farther and more often until you are able to walk *comfortably* for thirty to forty minutes daily.
3. If you want to increase your cardiovascular endurance, pick up your pace to a walk–jog or add a few hills to your route.
4. Walk heel first in order to minimize strain on the joints.
5. Wear good walking shoes and dress appropriately for the weather.
6. Listen to your body. Slow down or decrease your distance if you experience persistent fatigue or shortness of breath.

A LAST WORD

We are all aging. For too long, women have dreaded this part of their lives, feeling perhaps that they will have to give up control of their health and well-being when their bodies begin to age. On the contrary, we've just seen many ways we can enhance our later years, beginning with a lifelong commitment to exercise and good nutrition. There's a great sense of power and confidence when you know enough about your changing body to be able to make informed decisions and keep yourself healthy. With this knowledge, we can take the time to embrace our older selves, reflect on where we've been, and wonder where our journey may lead us.

S E V E N

CHOOSING AN ACTIVE LIFESTYLE

The self-help book seems like it's been with us forever, but actually, the idea of women making their own health and well-being a priority is relatively new. Throughout history, we as women have been expected to take care of everyone else's emotional and physical needs first. The families and communities that we tended assumed that we would always be there, mysteriously able to maintain good health in spite of adverse or stressful conditions. Only rarely did we admit that we were tired or ill. When you consider where we've been, you realize how revolutionary it is for us to suddenly be taking care of ourselves for a change.

For many of us, physical activity has become a major component of this new emphasis on self-care. An unprecedented amount of media attention has hailed exercise as a virtual cure-all for what ails us. And while some of the claims about exercise's beneficial effects are sensationalized, many are indeed true. Even so, some women still don't see physical activity as an answer for them personally.

Because many adult American women were not encouraged to be physically active as children, and have little experience with competition, they are hesitant to try something new. "I'd feel foolish," and "I know I won't be any good," are two of the most frequent responses women make when asked to take tennis lessons or join others for a game of golf. Another important barrier to exercise, identified as the most important by respondents to the Melpomene survey, was a lack of free time. Most women today find that time is precious; making time for yourself is difficult no matter what your age or circumstance.

In Melpomene's experience, most women have a hard time relating to the exercise books that have proliferated with the fitness boom. They call

us to ask, "I know it works for the actresses and young, thin, independently wealthy women, but how can physical activity help me feel better?
How can I fit it into my already busy schedule? How will I get started?
What will keep me motivated?" Certainly the physical benefits are a
strong motivator. In a 1984 Melpomene Institute membership study of
more than four hundred women, respondents were asked how important
they felt certain benefits of exercise were to them. The five benefits that
received the "most important" rating, and the percentage of women who
gave the rating were:

Cardiovascular fitness	82 percent
Improved muscle tone	82 percent
Firmer body	82 percent
Weight maintenance	78 percent
Improved self-image	70 percent

Some of the physical benefits of exercise mentioned above have been
well-documented in laboratory tests. The psychological gains are harder
to measure, however, and therefore have not been addressed as frequently
in research. In our study, women were able to offer direct feedback about
the personal growth they had experienced after becoming active. They
told us that exercise had changed their lives, personal relationships, and
self-esteem. It became apparent that women are exercising not only for a
healthier body but also for the good feelings that go hand-in-hand with
a physically active lifestyle.

SOCIAL BENEFITS OF EXERCISE

"It definitely has increased my social sphere and number of friends."

"I've met lots of good friends through orienteering."

"Physical activity has allowed me a vent for frustration and allowed
me fellowship and being part of a group."

The social interaction associated with exercise was a key psychological
benefit for many of the women in our membership study. This sentiment

has been echoed by thousands of women who have listened to our presentations, read our journal, or called us to get advice and share concerns. They felt that sports gave them a chance to meet new people, as well as a way to share a common activity with old friends. An interesting pattern emerged when women started commenting about the effects of exercise on their relationships. Many women noted that they had developed more tolerance and understanding toward others as a result of feeling better about themselves. Many relationships had improved or been sparked as a result of their new lifestyle. A surprising number had met their spouse or partner through a shared sport.

At the same time, some active women noticed that they no longer had as much time for sedentary friends, which may be because their new exercise programs were keeping them busy, or simply because they now had less in common with friends who had different lifestyle priorities.

"A shared activity with my spouse makes it more enjoyable; makes sure we both get our exercise each day."

"My husband, mother, and friends are very proud of my success in weight loss and physical abilities. I have more energy when I keep my weight down and get some *regular* activity."

"Since I feel better about myself, I deal with people and situations better. I have a firmer base."

IMPROVED SELF-ESTEEM

Improved self-image and confidence was a recurrent theme for participants in this and many other Melpomene studies. The confidence that comes from being able to do a sport successfully is a huge boost to self-esteem. The definition of success was different for each woman we interviewed. For some it meant swimming for ten minutes nonstop, and for others, it meant running a 26-mile marathon.

Our members also told us that they were proud to be participating or competing in a sport that society had at one time considered taboo or even impossible for women's participation. Like most of us, they had been programmed to believe that there were certain physical activities that they shouldn't or couldn't do because of their gender. Women who defy these damaging stereotypes gain confidence and a better self-image.

"I feel better about myself—my overall appearance. I have more confidence in myself, more self-assurance, and a better body image. I have something to talk about—myself."

"I have a better self-image, self-esteem. It's easier to love others when you love yourself."

"My improved self-image has made it easier on my family relationships."

"I feel better about my body. I am more outgoing, confident, and I take more risks."

A STRESS RELIEVER

For many, exercise was the best means they had found for relieving the day's stress and tensions. After working off the stress, the respondents in our membership study were left with that after-exercise "glow"—the feeling of more energy and well-being. Some said that the way they felt afterward was their main reason for exercising.

"I'm more relaxed."

"The best part of regular exercise is the feeling of exhilaration and well-being; always feeling energetic."

"Being in shape gives a feeling of well-being and confidence to take on challenges in all parts of life. Certainly I handle stress better."

"Exercise is very important to me as a means of stress management."

CHALLENGING YOURSELF

Finally, some of our members said that they valued physical activity because it offered them the chance to challenge themselves in the physical
arena. Through sport, they could set goals for themselves and experience
the sense of accomplishment that is so often lacking in our normal work
and home lives. Regardless of your age or ability, the chance to watch
yourself improve—to break your own records—can positively affect your
life.

If you have basically been sedentary, the first challenge is to decide
that physical activity and the lifestyle changes that usually accompany it
are worth the effort. Deciding to start and sticking with it may be two
different things, however. In short-term exercise programs, the dropout
rate is as high as 40 percent. In longer-term commitments (eight weeks
or more), that figure jumps to 75 percent.

STARTING AN EXERCISE PROGRAM

If you are not currently active, or wish to explore ways to increase or
diversify your level of physical activity, try filling out the personal profile
below. Analyzing your answers will give you some insights into your
knowledge and attitudes toward exercise.

A PERSONAL PROFILE

1. How many hours per day do you work (time that you do not consider
   leisure)?
2. How many hours per day are basically sitting work?
3. How many flights of stairs do you climb in an average week?
4. How many blocks do you walk in an average week?
5. How many hours per day do you spend doing housekeeping chores
   such as cooking and cleaning?
6. How many hours (or minutes) per day do you have that are "yours"?
   What do you do during this time (read, TV, knit, exercise)?
7. How interesting is physical activity to you (be honest!)?

8. What would be your main aims in beginning a physical activity program?
9. Think about your current schedule. What options do you have to fit in one-half hour, or one hour per day of exercise?
10. What does your body usually feel like at this time of day?
11. Are you more likely to exercise alone, with a friend, or in a class situation?
12. What are some realistic goals regarding physical activity for the next three weeks?
13. Try to list some goals for the next three months.

ANALYZING YOUR ANSWERS

Defining the number of hours you work is sometimes quite enlightening. We've used this questionnaire in many of our seminars, and invariably, women have been astounded by their own answers. "Well," sighed one. "No wonder I have such trouble finding time to exercise. I'm actually working a fifteen-hour day!" This woman is a public health administrator who works eight hours a day at the office and frequently brings home a briefcase of work that she tackles for two hours in the evening. In addition she is the mother of three young children who finds that the hours from 6 P.M. until they are in bed are filled with household responsibilities. On the other hand, one woman who has recently returned to school to complete a graduate degree found that for the first time she can actually attend classes and complete her studying in eight hours. "Until I filled out the profile, however," she remarked, "I was still living like I did when I worked full time and went to school. I realized I needed to figure out where the rest of my time was going."

More and more of us spend the better part of our day in work that is sedentary. Many of us have desk jobs that require little physical energy or effort. Most likely, we work in an environment where it is easier to take the elevator than use the stairs. Often, employees in these buildings would be hard-pressed to say where the stairway is located. Think of how inactive we've become in contrast to our ancestors who lived when farm, factory, and housework all required standing, lifting, and moving.

Because we are rarely forced to incorporate physical activity into our daily patterns, finding time to do so on a structured basis is often very difficult.

"When I get home, all I want to do is sit down with a drink!"

"I need to relax when I get home; going for a run would be ridiculous."

"What do you mean, take a break before dinner? If I did that, no one would eat until seven and that just wouldn't work."

To the people making these statements, the obstacles they list are real and seemingly insurmountable. If your answer to the question, How many hours per day do you have that are "yours"? is low, and you really treasure this time to read or watch TV, then it may be very hard to psychologically make the decision to begin exercising. Yet there is good evidence that if you can convince yourself that physical activity is important, you may indeed find a way to eliminate the obstacles. People who are not yet in the habit of exercising need a lot of evidence before they will believe that taking a brief, brisk walk or a leisurely jog will leave them more relaxed than sitting down with a drink or the evening paper. Scientific and practical observation proves this point. Ask any elementary schoolteacher who faces a classroom of kids in the afternoon. Students are always more alert and easier to teach after an active recess. After a lunch with no recess, the same students are more likely to feel like napping.

Carving out a time for exercise in an already busy day is a real problem for most of us. Thus, your answer to the question, How interesting is physical activity to you? is important. Many of us can think of physical activities that are not interesting to us at all. To some people, aerobic dance is ridiculous, while others think running looks like a modern-day form of torture. Naturally, choosing these activities would be self-defeating for such people; they'd have little incentive to overcome the inertia of their daily routine. The real key to choosing a physical activity or exercise program is to list four or five things that sound like fun and then find a sport that combines the best of these. Think of an activity that gave you pleasure when you were young, or that has intrigued you as an adult. "I'd really like to try racquetball," said one woman, "because it looks like fun."

Next, you might want to consider your answer to the question, What are your main aims in starting an exercise program? If your main aim is cardiovascular fitness, you should consider walking, running, vigorous biking, or swimming. Other programs will also qualify if you do them at least three times a week for a duration of thirty minutes at 80 percent of your heart rate.

If, however, your main aim is to look and feel better, you may be able to start at a lower level with sports that can be less demanding. Playing doubles tennis twice a week with other beginners may not improve your fitness level at first, but in time, as you become a better player, you may want to play more often or play a more vigorous game. (On the other hand, you might thoroughly enjoy your relaxed, nonstressful games and never make any great changes in intensity. That's completely up to you.)

Perhaps you want some variety and excitement in your exercise program. If you have primarily been a runner or a softball player for most of your life, it may be time to look at diversifying your activities. You may want to consider something entirely new like horseback riding, cross-country skiing, or golf.

Your choice of activity will also depend on your schedule and your need to be alone or with people. Lisa works with people all day. She frequently chairs meetings in the morning and spends all afternoon with clients. Her friend Chris urged her to join the local fitness club so that they could exercise together at the end of the day. Since Lisa was having trouble motivating herself to exercise, she decided to give it a try. The courts and track were well-maintained, the club was convenient, yet within two weeks, Lisa was ready to quit. What she hadn't realized was that the crowds that used the facility at the same time she did would put her on edge, especially after a full day of people contact. Instead, Lisa decided to tune up her old bike and strike out on her own.

Scheduling is particularly crucial where jobs and young children are involved. In a Melpomene Institute study of women who ran or swam during their pregnancies, a large number said that they exercised less and less after their child was born. One of the major reasons was not being able to find anyone to babysit. It's also hard for many women who work outside the home to justify leaving a child in daycare for an extra hour or two at the end of a day. For this reason many chose to exercise before others were awake. Jane frequently is at the YWCA pool by 6 A.M. "It's my only choice," she says, "and while I almost resented it at first, I've discovered it's a great way to start the day." It's not as easy to find a partner for tennis at that hour, but groups of runners and bikers are also known to meet, exercise, shower, and be at work by 8 A.M. Scheduling may pose more problems if you decide to set a time-consuming goal like running a marathon or riding a century (a 100-mile bike ride).

What happens if your body is not ready to exercise at the hour that's most convenient for you? If you're like Mary, you wake up feeling as if you are fifty-nine instead of thirty-six. Mary has some mild arthritis that only bothers her early in the morning. She finds that lunchtime or after work, though they may not be as convenient, are better times for her to exercise.

It is clear from these brief examples that choosing an exercise program can be more complex than promoters would have us believe. The ads look great: young, attractive, thin people swimming and hitting tennis balls as if there are no hassles involved. While most people who are serious about physical exercise know that it's not always convenient or easy, they are also the first to attempt to convince you to give it a try.

For many women, just deciding to become physically active can be the biggest hurdle to overcome. Some women are able to begin by just walking out the front door to a regular walking or running program. If you are like most women, however, there are many practical considerations to make before starting. Your situation is unique—and only you can determine what will work given your lifestyle, time constraints, and level of commitment. We offer the following suggestions and encouragement to anyone trying to become more active.

Consider Your Health. Each woman needs to take stock of her health and medical history before entering an exercise program of any kind. Some general guidelines established by the American College of Sports Medicine suggest that if you are under age thirty-five with no history of cardiovascular problems or other risk factors, you need not get a medical checkup.

You may, however, choose to check with your healthcare provider if you have concerns about your health or the exercise program you are about to undertake. We encourage you to make an appointment if you have an underlying medical condition such as cardiovascular disease, hypertension, or diabetes, or if you have a family history of any of these conditions.

There are other health factors that you will want to take into consideration before starting to exercise, including any chronic conditions or illnesses, disabilities, or previous injuries. These things shouldn't stop you from being physically active, but you should consider them when choosing your sport or the kind of equipment you will use.

Choose the Right Physical Activity for Yourself. There are many factors to keep in mind when you choose an activity. The most important, however, is that it should be fun. If you are not enjoying your exercise program or the sport you choose, you will not continue to do it. Ideally, you will be able to find a few activities that you enjoy well enough to keep you active throughout your lifetime.

Your age might be a factor in the activity you choose. Our membership survey of more than four hundred women showed us that favored activities do seem to change with age. Running, for example, was extremely popular with women in their forties and younger, but quickly lost its allure for women in their fifties, sixties, and above. The popularity of walking and hiking, however, rose dramatically for women in their sixties and seventies. Playing golf also became more popular as age increased. After age fifty, the number of women working out with weights or playing team activities, racquetball, or squash dropped to zero.

While age is not necessarily a barrier to any activity, it seems that as the women in this study grew older, they gravitated toward different sports that fit their changing needs. This change in choice of activity with age reminds us once again that sport is a treat for the self, and should be a source of enjoyment and relaxation.

The time you have for physical activity may also influence your choice of activity. If your time is limited, as is the case for many of us, you may choose a daily activity that can be done in a fairly short amount of time, and save more time-consuming activities for the weekends. For example, you may take a walk each day during the week and plan to canoe for several hours on the weekend.

A full calendar of family/friend responsibilities and/or work may force you to come up with creative ways to squeeze in workouts during the week, which may mean a tennis game during lunch hour or trading child-care with another physically active friend. If you have younger children, look for a health club that offers childcare. Once they get older, your kids may enjoy a swim or dribbling the basketball at the "Y" while you attend exercise class.

Your environment, including climate, community, and available facilities, can also affect your choice of physical activity. A northern climate may not seem like an obvious deterrent to your biking program in May, but just wait until December and January roll around. You may be forced to switch to another sport for the winter, or perhaps find a facility where you can exercise indoors during the coldest days. The community you live in may also shape the activity you choose. If you live in a large city, it may take longer to get to safe, wide-open roads than it would if you lived in a rural setting. Some rural settings, however, may not offer the kind of equipment or facilities you need for your chosen sport. Considerations like these can be especially crucial if you travel a lot. Finding an alternate activity that you can "take with you" might be to your advantage.

For almost any activity that needs an actual facility such as a pool, ice rink, court, or weight room, you will need to spend some time shopping for a club that will suit your needs. Some things you'll want to consider before joining are the initiation and monthly fees, the financial stability of the club, the number of other members, the equipment available for your activity, locker and shower facilities, the instructors' qualifications, the hours, and the location. If the club is far from your home, try to imagine yourself getting home from work and then getting back in the car to commute to your club. Would it be a deterrent?

Many physical activities don't require the use of a facility, but almost all require some special equipment or clothing. This expense, be it large or small, may influence your decision to get involved in an activity. For example, if you were to choose a walking program, you'd need only a good pair of shoes. If you want to start cycling, however, the start-up costs would certainly be higher. We recommend that you list the clothing, equipment, and facility costs associated with your sport before deciding to make a firm commitment. Also, consider borrowing equipment instead of buying until you are sure you like the activity. Once you've participated for a while, you'll also have a better idea of what style of equipment suits you best.

Finally, before you undertake a new exercise program, do some soul searching to find out what kind of a participant you'll be. Are you likely to continue a program without group support or will you need the camaraderie of an organized class? Will you participate on the hottest or coldest days of the year or do you need an indoor alternative? Are you bored easily? Do you need several different activities to keep you involved? Knowing what motivates and excites you will be important a few months down the road, when the novelty of the sport has worn off, and you might be tempted to stop exercising.

Have a Plan. Writing down what you need before you go to the grocery store always seems to speed the trip and keeps you from buying things you don't need. In the same way, an exercise plan is a good idea when you are beginning to be physically active. An example of a plan may be a cycling schedule that will allow you to train for a one-hundred mile bike ride in eight weeks. There will be a set mileage and intensity for each day, as well as special days for hill work or fast sprinting to build strength. Another example of a plan might be to walk around the block every day for a week, with a goal of being able to finish the walk without feeling tired. Whatever your ambitions are, a plan will provide you with a sensible program and will help you stay committed to that program.

There are several ways to go about finding the right plan for yourself in the activity you choose. Health clubs or the local YWCA offer classes in many activities from aerobics to swimming to weight lifting. There are also many clubs formed by local people who like to get together to share their sport. The best place to find out about these clubs is at a local store that sells equipment in that sport. For example, if you were trying to hook up with a woman's cycling group, you might try asking a woman bike mechanic where she rides. Members of these clubs can give you tips as well as encouragement as you become accustomed to exercise.

Books can also be a valuable source of information when you're setting up a plan. Remember, however, that you will not get feedback from a book if you have specific questions or problems once you begin. There are two types of books that offer advice on exercise plans. One kind will offer you a very specific, day-by-day plan that you can follow easily. The other will be more general, offering enough information for you to make your own program. In the bibliography section at the end of this book, we have listed some references that we have found to be helpful.

Some of you won't need or want any outside direction. Your goal—to walk three days a week or take tennis lessons—may be something you can do quite independently. Sometimes, however, having a friend know about, or share, that goal can be very helpful. Ellen and Frances insist they would not have succeeded in their goal of becoming more physically active without each other. Ellen asked Frances one day if she would be interested in walking a mile or so several days a week. Frances agreed and remarked that she had actually been thinking about getting more exercise since she retired. The critical decision, although they didn't realize it at the time, was to meet on a street corner midway between their homes. "The first day it rained," remembers Frances. "I sat by my phone waiting for Ellen to call and say she wanted to cancel." Ellen of course was waiting for Frances to be the first to call. Since neither of them wanted to be the first to break the plan, each went out in the mild rain. "The secret," says Ellen, "was meeting at the corner. It meant that we were serious about walking. If we had met at one of our homes, I'm sure there would have been days when we would have stayed in and had a cup of coffee instead."

Go Slowly. Once you have convinced yourself that you will be physically active, you are probably eager to get started, which is good. Hold onto that enthusiasm; you may need it in a few months when time pressures tempt you to quit. Right now, however, our advice is to go slowly. Overdoing physical activity in the early stages of a program is an invitation to burnout and injury. There will be many opportunities to push yourself, but right now, taking it easy will help you to stay fresh and committed to your new activity.

Stick with It! Promise yourself a minimum amount of time to try your new program. Eight weeks is a good length to give you an idea of whether this is the right plan or activity for you. Any less than five or six weeks is not enough time to make a fair judgment. Also, the longer you keep with a plan, the more the activity becomes a habit and a regular part of your life.

There will be days when you don't feel like working out. That's okay— we all have those days. Remember that you are making a major change in your life and it may not be easy. Some small rewards might help you stick to your plan on those days when exercise is particularly tough. (You'll find more on staying motivated in the next section.)

Have Fun! Again, it is important that you are having fun in your exercise program. There are many tricks to keep yourself motivated, but if the activity is not initially fun for you to do, you will not keep with it. You may have to try a few different sports until you find one or two that you really enjoy. Don't give up—physical activity *is* fun!

STAYING MOTIVATED

Perhaps one of the hardest parts of regular physical activity is staying motivated so that you exercise on a regular basis. Often boredom or increased time constraints are enough of a roadblock to make you stop exercising altogether.

As part of our second membership survey conducted in 1984, we asked respondents, "What do you consider the worst part of regular physical activity?" Their responses were diverse, but the overall theme was the same: The biggest challenge is to stay motivated enough to do physical activity regularly.

"Exercise can become another thing on an endless list to do."

"The hardest part is finding the time."

"Getting my bones out of bed and out the door is the worst part."

"The toughest thing is deciding to do it each day."

". . . boredom . . ."

". . . bad weather . . ."

We also asked respondents in the 1984 membership survey to rank which obstacles were most likely to keep them from exercising. As you can see by looking at the table below, time is the largest barrier for many women trying to maintain an active lifestyle.

EXPERIENCED OBSTICLES TO PHYSICAL ACTIVITY

%	Obstacle
52.9%	Not enough time due to job
39.7%	Not enough time due to family responsibilities
20.5%	Fear that I wouldn't do well
18.4%	Lack of encouragement
18.2%	None
17.9%	People believing I shouldn't be athletic
15.4%	Shower, fix hair, etc. after exercise
10.3%	People believing I couldn't be athletic
7.3%	Ridicule
7.3%	Monetary concerns
7.3%	Conflicts about role of physical activity

With all these barriers to regular physical activity, you might wonder how so many women manage to overcome the obstacles and remain motivated. Deep-down faith in the results helps, but that's not always enough to rouse us from our recliners. Below are some tactics and ideas you might try if you are finding yourself with more than your share of excuses about why you shouldn't get out there and do your activity.

Do It with Someone Else. Many of the women in our survey said that one of the best parts of physical activity is the chance to exercise with friends or family members, as well as the chance to meet new friends. There are several ways to find people who share your interests. You can start by attending an event or a race in your activity. Ask the participants about clubs or teams in your area; if there are none, you could even try starting one! Talk about your sport at work, at church, or wherever your find yourself; eventually you are bound to bump into someone who shares your enthusiasm and has been looking for a partner. If you're interested in taking up a new activity, you could create a built-in partner by asking a friend to take lessons with you.

Try a Change. If you find yourself bored with your exercise routine, try a change. It doesn't have to be big; you can alter your route, work out at a different time, or, if you live in the north country, you could do your sport indoors in the winter. For some women, changing the structure of their exercise routine can bring freshness back. For example, if you are swimming a mile in the pool every other day, throwing in some sets of fast laps, arms only, or kicking only, may make your mile like a new workout.

Perhaps you need to switch or add a new sport to your physical activity program. A day or two a week on your bike or in the pool can be effective in perking up a stale running schedule. Also, seasonal changes offer many opportunities for change in your program. Winter sports such as cross-country skiing or snowshoeing can give you ample exercise while enhancing your overall conditioning. Swimming, aerobics, or walking around a track can also be substituted when it is too hot to run or play tennis outdoors. By treating yourself to something new, you get to try other sports or different variations of your own sport to see what works, what you like, and what you may want to add to your regular program in the future.

Give Yourself a Reward. When you are feeling sluggish, offer yourself a treat for completing your workout. You might promise yourself a long hot bath, a massage, a new piece of sport clothing, or whatever really pleases you. This reward is your way of patting yourself on the back. Not only will you feel proud of yourself for having completed your workout but you'll have a reward to look forward to as well.

Set Goals. Goals can be wonderful incentives to continue with an exercise program. Your goal can be a future competition in your activity, keeping with it for a set number of months, or obtaining a certain level of endurance or skill. Be realistic with your goals. The goals you set should be obtainable for you, yet feel like an achievement. Don't set marks so high that you will never be able to obtain them; doing so will set you up for failure and work against your efforts to stay motivated.

Get Into or Out of Competition. If you are competitive in your sport, give yourself a break and do your sport just for fun. Without the pressure of upcoming competitions, you'll be able to recapture the sense of fun that first attracted you to the activity.

On the other hand, if you have never competed in your sport, you may want to set your sights on an upcoming event or competition. If you are not feeling competitive, there are often events held in various activities that are noncompetitive gatherings. For example, organized bike rides, fun runs, or exhibitions in various sports can fit into this category. An upcoming event in your sport may give you a tangible reason for keeping up with your physical activity program.

Try Something Completely New. Have you always wanted to snowshoe? Do you wonder what whitewater canoeing is like? Have you been itching to try a mountain bike? Now is the time to give these and other interesting activities a try. These days, you can rent almost any piece of sporting equipment imaginable. You may want to get a friend or a group of friends to try a new activity with you. You have nothing to lose and everything to gain—you may end up with a new favorite pastime!

Set Up a Home Fitness Center. A home fitness center does not have to be a weight room and exercise studio. It can be as simple as an aerobics tape and a good mat or a stationary exercise bike. Think of your home equipment as a backup for those rainy days or the days when you don't have the time to get out of the house. A ten-second commute to your basement will leave you plenty of time to exercise, even when you have less than an hour. Your home equipment might also be an alternative to your regular routine, just for the sake of variety!

Avoid Becoming Obsessive About Exercise. For many women, exercise can bring on feelings of compulsion, with subsequent guilt if they skip a day or want to stop for a while. Some of the women in the Melpomene Institute membership survey mentioned this obsession with exercise as a negative part of being active.

"It can become so important that it begins to assume too much priority."

"The worst part of exercise is the pressure to do it regularly and the disappointment on the days when I just can't discipline myself to do it."

"Exercise can be obsessively burdensome at times."

"Having guilt feelings if you miss a day is a negative."

"I tend to become so obsessed that I risk injury from overdoing it."

Experts in sports psychology debate whether physical activity is an addiction, and if so, whether it is a positive or a negative addiction. Certainly, we all have days when we push ourselves out the door to exercise, or feel disappointed in ourselves for having missed a workout. If exercise begins to bring about strong obsessive feelings, however, it may be time to take a break or switch physical activities.

Review Your Progress. Keep an informal journal or jot notes on a calendar so that you can look back at what you were doing six months ago, even when you first started to become physically active. Your progress will surprise you and give you a reason to pat yourself on the back. Also, when you see how far you have come, it will be tougher to quit your program from lack of motivation. Your progress and milestones, however large or small, are cause to celebrate!

Build Fitness Into Other Areas of Your Life. If you find yourself without the time or motivation to do your regular workout, look for creative ways to turn your everyday activities into pulse-quickening exercise. For example, leave your car in the driveway and ride your bike or walk to work. Look for the stairs in your building and use them. If you are homebound with children, build some activity around exercise, like a soccer game or a stroll in the park. Some household chores can give you the benefits of aerobic exercise without taking the time to change into sweats or drive to the gym. Some possibilities include vigorous spring cleaning, shoveling snow, gardening, or doing yardwork.

Take Some Time Off. Sluggishness and a lack of desire to exercise can be signs that you are doing more than you should, either mentally or physically. Your body may be telling you to take a break, or at least to back off for a while. When it's time to start exercising again, your body will let you know. You will find yourself missing your physical activity and wanting to move. Taking a break can bring a sense of novelty and enthusiasm back to your workouts.

AVOIDING INJURY

Becoming injured is a very real concern for many physically active women. Fifteen percent of the women in our membership survey said that injuries and aches and pains were the worst part of regular exercise.

"Some days are just bad; I seem to injure easily."

"The worst part of exercise is having to lay off because of injuries."

"One year ago I sustained tibial stress fractures. I am still recovering from this injury and have to take it easy."

"I have sore legs from concrete and pavement."

Some injuries, especially those from overuse, can be avoided with some common sense. Although we all overdo it sometime, it is important to take care of our most important piece of equipment—our bodies!

Here are some guidelines Melpomene offers to help women avoid injury:

Warm Up Before You Exercise. Before you start moving your body, take time to stretch. Stretching loosens the muscles you are about to use and increases your range of motion. Inflexible, "cold" muscles are more prone to injury from pulls and strains. Stretching should be a permanent part of your program, not just a a quick fix if you think you are becoming injured.

Start Your Physical Activity Slowly. By starting slowly, you are allowing your body to warm up, your muscles to loosen, and your heart rate and breathing to gradually accelerate.

Slow Down and Cool Off After Exercise. Walking or doing light stretching is a good way to end your activity. Cooling down allows your heart rate and breathing to return to normal (pre-exercise) levels. Also stretching after your workout will help you to avoid muscle soreness.

Use the Proper Equipment for Your Activity. Your sports equipment should fit you well, be in good working order, and be comfortable. Ill-fitting equipment, from shoes to bicycles, can be a primary cause of sports injuries. We feel that getting good equipment is making an investment in yourself. If your equipment is uncomfortable or broken, you open yourself not only to injury, but also to discouragement. You may not perform as well or have as much fun as your would with reliable equipment, and consequently, you may not choose to participate in that sport again. Although we suggest good equipment, it does not have be the most expensive, top-of-the-line piece of equipment you can find. By reading magazines in your chosen sport, visiting professionally staffed stores, and trying out various brands, you should be able to make an educated, cost-effective choice. A word of caution here: Even if you are borrowing equipment, or trying out different brands, fit is still important.

Be sure to check out the new lines of sport equipment that are specially sized and designed for women, including bikes, running shoes, ski boots, and weight machines. These products have been a real boon, particularly for smaller women who have a hard time finding men's equipment that will fit them. Cyclists under 5′4″, for instance, can now find bikes with a smaller front wheel and a shorter top tube so they can reach the handlebars comfortably. While we are encouraged by this trend, and hope that it continues, we continue to urge women to be cautious buyers. Be aware that some women's equipment is still not as well designed as men's equipment. A classic case is the mixte bicycle frame that has a downward sloping top tube rather than a horizontal one (presumably so you can wear a skirt when you ride). Structurally, mixte frames are not as strong as men's diamond-shaped frames, and have been known to break under pressure. In cases like these, buy the best equipment available as long as you can find the right fit for you.

Be Consistent with Your Exercise Program. Check the waiting room of any sports medicine clinic on Monday morning, and you're likely to find a good number of achy weekend athletes. Take the woman, for example, who plays tennis every other weekend and then heads for the ski slopes for a week of all-day, everyday activity. Even though she is regularly active, her body is not primed for this intensity or type of activity. If she had been doing strengthening exercises, or perhaps bicycling consistently for a few months before the trip, she may have been less prone to injury.

In any sport, the best way to avoid injury is to set up and maintain a program that balances all three aspects of physical conditioning: strength, flexibility, and endurance. An aerobics class that begins with stretching, moves into aerobic movement and strengthening exercises, and ends with stretching again, is a good example of a balanced workout.

If you want to maintain fitness, physical activity should become part of your lifestyle for at least a half-hour three days a week. Also, you will receive more benefits from your exercise program if you do it every other day, rather than three days in a row.

Listen to Your Body. Your body will tell you when it is worn down or getting injured, but it is also important for you to know your limits. If you are becoming fatigued, a day off from your exercise program may be just what you need. Also, think twice about exercising when you are getting sick. Physical activity may make you feel better mentally, but it may prolong or aggravate a cold or illness. If you are running a fever, plan on resting.

Your body will also tell you if your are getting injured. Pain, sleeplessness, irritability, fatigue, or slower reflexes are signs that you are overtraining or just getting stale. You body is sending you the message to take it easy for a while.

Don't Overdo It. This rule is especially important for women who are beginning an exercise program. Often our enthusiasm will push us to do more than our bodies can manage. For example, it is not realistic to think you can run a marathon three months after starting a running program.

Increase the Intensity and Duration of Your Physical Activity Gradually. Adding a little more each time you exercise is a sensible way to reach your fitness goals. If you are making a change in your exercise pattern, incorporate that change slowly. If you decide to add speed intervals to your swimming program, for example, add a few intervals at a time until you reach your desired number of sets. You may also want to take an easy swim, go for a walk, or rest the following day.

Rest. Rest is as important to your fitness program as any other aspect. On the days you rest, your muscles recover from the exertion of your previous activity. The more strenuous your physical activity, the greater the need for you to rest. If you participate in more than one sport, it is possible to rest in one sport by doing another. For example, if bicycling is your primary sport, a restful day might be an easy swim in a nearby lake.

Pay Attention to Weather Conditions. If you exercise out-of-doors, weather can greatly affect your workouts. For example, if you are planning a long bicycle ride and find it is 40° F and raining, you may choose to postpone or alter your ride. If you do choose to do the long ride, you will need to dress appropriately and take along a change of clothes. Similarly, if you are planning your weekly running speed workout for noon when it is 98° F, you may consider postponing it.

Adapting to weather includes dressing properly for both temperature and weather conditions. In cold weather, dressing in layers of clothing keeps you warmer than one or two heavy articles, because air warmed by your body heat becomes trapped in between layers of clothing, keeping you warm longer. If it is cold and windy, you will want to include an outer layer of wind-breaking fabric, like nylon, Gore-Tex, or Thintech, or other breathable fabric. It is especially important to wear a hat in cold weather, because much of your body heat is lost through the top of your head.

On windy days, you may want to think about the prevailing wind direction before you set your course. If you head into the wind on a run, bike ride, or cross-country ski, the wind will be at your back when you turn around to come home. You will feel a bit warmer, and the wind will gently push you on your way. If the wind is at your back when your start, you will find yourself fighting the wind all the way home. Winds also have a peculiar way of becoming stronger and colder in the afternoon, when you are most apt to start tiring. Precipitation is another element you'll learn to respect if you spend much time out-of-doors. Even a warm rain can chill you if you become soaked to the skin. Don't forget to pack a waterproof or water-resistant outer layer if the skies are threatening rain or snow.

If you are exercising in hot weather, drinking large amounts of liquids is the best way to help your body cool itself. If you fail to drink enough during extended exercise in hot weather, you can become dehydrated, causing heat stroke or heat exhaustion. Some danger signals are:

- Light-headedness
- Dizziness
- Clamminess
- Lack of perspiration
- Shivering
- Feeling cold

If you or someone you are with is experiencing any of these symptoms in hot weather, get to a shady or cool spot immediately and seek medical help. Overheating can be life threatening!

Experts disagree as to what is the best liquid for athletes to drink in hot weather. Some believe the plain water is best because it empties quickly from the stomach and is utilized quickly by the body. Proponents of sports drinks feel that the added electrolytes in these drinks replace the electrolytes your body loses through sweating. Whatever you choose to drink during hot-weather exercise, be sure to drink before you start, during the activity, and after you finish.

Clothes for hot-weather workouts should be light and comfortable. If you tend to perspire a lot, you may want to avoid cotton because it absorbs sweat and becomes heavy and uncomfortable. Instead, you may be better off with clothes made of polypropylene or a similar fiber that wicks moisture away from your body so it can be quickly evaporated into the air. Don't forget the parts of your skin that are exposed; sunscreen is a must if you are in the sun for long periods of time.

Know the Signs of Impending Overuse Injury. We all know we're hurt when we have a traumatic injury like a sprained ankle or a twisted knee, but overuse injuries from exercise can be sneaky. If may be difficult to know if you are really injured or just suffering the common aches, pains, and sore muscles that accompany an active lifestyle.

Some common signs of an overuse injury can be:

- *Pain.* Joint pain or pain when you touch a specific site can be a sign of trouble. Throbbing pain hours after a workout may indicate impending injury.
- *Swelling.* Swelling is obvious in some injuries, but in others the area may just feel swollen without changing in size. It may help to compare the size and the sensitivity of that body part to the same part on the other side.
- *Reduced range of motion.* You may have an overuse injury if you are limited in movement in a muscle or joint when compared to the other side, or if you detect weakness. For instance, if you are favoring a leg because you feel your knee might "go out," you may be overdoing it.

Know How to Treat an Overuse Injury. There are several things you can do if you have an overuse injury, or if you suspect you might be injured:

- Stop doing any activity that causes you pain or that seems to aggravate your injury. You may want to seek medical help if you think the injury is traumatic enough.
- Rest the injured part of your body.
- If there is swelling from your injury, you will want to keep it to a minimum. There are a few ways to reduce swelling:

  Ice the injury for the first twenty-four to forty-eight hours. Crushed ice or a soft ice pack works best because you can mold it around the injured body part. It is important to note that heat will not reduce swelling; instead, heat actually increases blood flow and swelling.

  Use compression to keep the swelling down, which is done by wrapping the injured area with an Ace bandage. Although you want to limit circulation, be careful not to wrap it so tightly that circulation is completely cut off from that area.

  Elevate the injured part of the body to help keep swelling down.
- You may choose to switch sports for a while until your injury heals. Be sure the activity you substitute doesn't further stress your injury. For example, if you have shin pain from your aerobics class, changing to running will not give your shins a break. Instead, you would want a sport that is nonjarring, such as cycling or swimming.
- You will want to seek medical treatment if the injury is still painful several days later, if swelling persists, if range of motion is severely limited, or if your injury has lasted more than a week or two with rest.

GUIDELINES FOR SPECIFIC SPORTS

AEROBIC DANCE

Martha Stoll Albertson, an exercise physiologist at The Marsh, a Center for Health and Balance, in Minnetonka, Minnesota, offers this information on aerobic dance.

BENEFITS

1. Increases aerobic capacity.
2. Lowers weight and blood pressure.
3. Increases flexibility.
4. Tones muscles.
5. Builds self-esteem.

GETTING STARTED

1. The motivation for taking an aerobics class should come from you, not from your friends, relatives, or co-workers. Your heart must be in the plan in order to stick to it.

2. Consult your physician if you plan to begin an aerobic exercise program, especially if you're over thirty-five or if you now have a fairly sedentary lifestyle. If you have any cardiac risk, factors, such as high blood pressure, high cholesterol, smoking, familial history of cardiac incidents, or diabetes, an exercise stress test may be prescribed.

3. Be choosy when considering exercise or activity classes. Check with various agencies and facilities to find out what kind of training their instructors have received. Ask if you can "test-drive" a class before signing up. If you are completely fatigued after the trial class, it may be too advanced for you. You should feel invigorated, not spent.

4. Select an aerobic exercise class that you enjoy. You have individual fitness needs. The class should match your present fitness level and include the following elements: a warm-up, cardiovascular training, flexibility and muscle toning components, and a cool-down. The warm-up and cool-down are especially important.

5. Fashionable clothing is not necessary. All you need is comfortable clothing and aerobics shoes that support both lateral and front/back movement.

6. Start your exercise program gradually, with a low impact class, if possible. It pays to take beginning classes at first so you can get the hang of the routines. Nothing is more frustrating than not being able to keep up with the class because you're not familiar with the basic moves.

1. Another key to enjoying your aerobic class is to keep your competitive nature out of the studio. Concentrate on what is safe and healthy for you.

2. The old adage "no pain, no gain" can be a dangerous one. Your aerobic exercise class should not leave you in pain.

3. Establish goals, don't make any excuses, exercise with a friend, and above all make it fun! The end product should be a stronger, healthier, more flexible, and vital *you.*

BICYCLING

Megan Webster, a United States Cycling Federation racer, and former Minnesota State Women's Cycling Champion, provided this information.

1. Adjust your seat so you are not too high or too low from the pedals. Even an inch can put undue stress on your knees. To find the proper height for your seat, have a friend stand behind you and watch your pedal. The seat should be low enough so that your hips don't shift from side to side as you pedal. When your leg is at the bottom of the stroke, it should be slightly bent at the knee. Anther way to measure height is to put your heel on the pedal and fully extend your leg. In this position, your leg should be almost straight, with no bend in the knee.

2. Make sure you are not too stretched out or cramped on your bike. It's natural for your shoulders and neck to hurt on the first few rides of the season, but if it continues, visit your local bike shop. Ask them about changing the length of your handlebar stem, moving your seat back or forth, or tilting the seat up a bit.

3. If you are saddle sore, try wearing a good pair of cycling shorts with a real chamois or synthetic chamois padding. They are meant to be worn without underwear. If these shorts don't help, look into buying a new seat. Saddles come in a variety of widths, and some are now made with a gel material that cushions the pressure points.

4. Always wear a helmet. Even the best riders are victims of motorists' mistakes.

5. Wear well-padded cycling gloves and alternate between three hand positions: on top of the handlebars, over the brake hoods, and on the bottom of the bars.

GETTING IN SHAPE

1. Keep your cadence high (60 to 100 revolutions per minute) and bend your elbows slightly to decrease stress on your joints.

2. Ride five or six days a week. Alternate hard days with easy days. On "hard" days do either the speed, power, or hill workout below. On "easy" days ride a comfortable distance at a lively pace.

3. Find a group of people to ride with who are at your level or a little better. Each week, increase the speed and distance of your ride.

GETTING BETTER

Here are some sample workouts to help you improve various aspects of your biking performance:

1. *Speed.* Sprint 200 yards at top speed, recover completely, and repeat until your form or speed begin to decline.

2. *Endurance.* Do one long ride each week, increasing the length weekly. Keep the pace snappy. A long, slow ride does not result in improvement.

3. *Power.* In a high gear, stand up and ride for several minutes. Recover to a heart rate of 70 percent of maximum and do five or six times. Or do decreasing intervals of 2, 1.5, 1, and 0.5 minute, letting your heart recover to 70 percent between each one.

4. *Hill climbing.* Ride a few hills each time you go out. Find a two- or three-minute hill and give it your all five or six times, pacing yourself to keep a steady momentum all the way to the top. Shift into a low gear at the bottom of the hill and "spin" until you meet the resistance of the hill.

5. *Form.* Have another cyclist check to see that your back is flat when

you are in a crouched position. Try to pedal with only one leg in order to find and eliminate the dead spots in your revolution.

CROSS-COUNTRY SKIING

Long time cross-country skier and Melpomene president Judy Lutter has this advice on this exhilerating winter sport.

BENEFITS

1. Excellent aerobic conditioning exercise.
2. Uses most of your major muscle groups.
3. Injuries are rare.
4. One of the most pleasurable sports.
5. Provides a seasonal sport alternative.

EQUIPMENT TIPS

1. *Touring cross-country skis.* These versatile skis are intended for diagonal-stride (Nordic) skiing. They come in either waxable or waxless styles. The difference is that waxless skis can be used without having to prepare the bottom surfaces with waxes. In place of wax, plastic "fish-scales" on the bottom of the ski grip the snow in almost any weather condition. The disadvantage is that waxless skis are not very fast. If you plan to ski often during a winter, you will probably want to consider the faster waxable skis, even though you will have to "wax up" before you head out. Contrary to popular belief, the waxing process does not have to be complex, and it will give you a quicker, more responsive glide than you can get with most waxless skis.

2. *Skating skis.* Skating skis are designed specifically for a technique called skating that has become popular within the last five years. The skating ski is stiffer, has a built-up sidewall, and is shorter. It is helpful to have all skis professionally fitted to your particular height, weight, and type of skiing, but when you are buying skating skis, fit is especially important. Skating skis start at about $100 and can go as high as $400.

3. *Boots.* Boots for skating skis are generally higher in order to provide

more ankle support. Ski boots range in price from $65 to $300. A beginning skier can generally start at the bottom end of the price range and expect equipment to last for many years.

4. *Poles.* Poles also vary in price and strength depending on use. Skating poles are longer, stronger, and more expensive. Again it is important to have ski poles that fit your height and anticipated use.

5. *Fanny pack.* Many people wear a small fanny pack when skiing that holds some snacks, lip balm, sun protection, and water. Cross-country skiing any distance will usually cause you to sweat, so it is a good idea to drink before you start as well as during your ski to prevent dehydration.

GETTING STARTED

1. Dressing correctly is a key to comfort. An ideal temperature range for cross-country skiing is from 10° F to 22° F, but since most skiers will only find a few ideal days per season, it is important to know how to dress for any weather. For the most part, people tend to overdress. In addition to considering factors such as wind, snow, sun, or clouds, your pace and intensity of skiing will also influence how much you should wear. Remember that you will be using your whole body, and will most likely warm up quickly. Wearing layered clothing that you can remove and put in your pack is an excellent idea. If the weather is below 10° F, it is smart to wear some sort of polypropylene product, which will wick water away from your body and keep you warmer. Remember to wear a hat in colder weather and to have a face mask if the weather is below zero. Warm gloves or mittens are another important requirement. Ski boots now are lined with an insulating inner liner, but wool socks are a must. Lightweight polypropylene socks to be worn under the wool socks are also a good idea for particularly cold weather. It is also possible to buy a bootie, which goes over your boot and adds further warmth for particularly cold days.

2. Consider taking lessons. While diagonal-stride skiing is a fairly easy technique to master, we recommend that we rent skis for your first try and get a lesson at the same time. The hints provided by a good instructor will make skiing far more pleasurable. Most people who decide to try the

skating method also take at least one lesson. While it may look easy, a few subtle directions and techniques make it much more efficient and fun.

3. Golf courses and parks are a good place to start skiing and an increasing number of parks now provide skis for rental at a reasonable rate. Almost all ski areas will have well-marked trails that will also let you know degree of difficulty. An "easiest" trail may vary in difficulty among geographical regions of the United States, so it is smart to ask some specifics about the trail. Most trail systems will also have the length of the trail marked so you can judge how long you will be out.

GETTING BETTER

1. Try some intermediate and eventually some advanced trails. However, don't get into situations that will be frustratingly difficult or even dangerous. Ask someone at the warming hut or visitor center to describe the trail conditions before you head out.

2. Try racing. Cross-country ski racing is gaining in popularity across the United States. Look for races in your local paper or see if there is a ski club in your area. Many races have five- or ten-year age divisions. Distances for cross-country ski races vary greatly from 5 kilometers to the famous Birkebeiner held every year in Hayward, Wisconsin, which is 55 kilometers in length. Terrain and weather conditions mean it is much harder to predict your time on a course, but competitive women in their twenties area able to ski a 10 kilometer in twenty-nine minutes; excellent times for women in their forties are in the thirty-five-minute range.

SWIMMING

Swim coach and current masters swimmer Sharon Simpson offers the following on swimming.

BENEFITS

1. Is an excellent way to develop cardiorespiratory fitness.
2. Uses most of the major muscle groups.
3. Is continuous in nature and can be done at a moderate pace.

4. Injuries are rare because swimming puts less stress on joints and muscles than weight-bearing exercises do (water buoys you up!).
5. Can be enjoyed throughout one's lifetime, both leisurely or competitively.
6. Can be done individually, with a friend, or with a group.

EQUIPMENT TIPS

1. Swimsuits: Nylon adds durability to a suit, and Lycra adds comfort. Both are important if you intend to swim regularly.

2. If you haven't used goggles before, we recommend that you take time to find some that are comfortable and that fit your face. Goggles improve vision and reduce eye irritation. They allow you to see where you are going, monitor your arm action, and generally make swimming more enjoyable. Goggles come in a variety of colors and shapes to fit anyone, but they require a period of adjustment. After about a week of making minor adjustments to the nosepiece and the sides, they'll fit you like a glove and you won't want to swim without them. If fogging is a problem, try using a defogging solution, or buy nonfogging goggles.

GETTING STARTED

1. Consider taking lessons. With basic training, anyone can learn to swim or learn to swim more efficiently. Check with your local community swimming program, the YMCA/YWCA, local high schools or colleges, or a nearby health club. You can usually choose either group instruction or private lessons.

2. Find a pool that has scheduled times for adults to swim laps, and that uses lane lines (on the bottom of the pool) to separate the swimmers into groups.

3. Check with the lifeguard regarding lane pace at your pool. Most lap swim programs have slow, medium, and fast lanes. Also check the circle pattern, which establishes the direction of travel around the black lines on the bottom of the pool. You will swim up one side of the line and down the other, going clockwise or counterclockwise, depending on the

rules at your pool. When you are just beginning, choose the slow lanes and stop at each end of the pool, stopping at the corner to let other swimmers pass by.

4. Start slow and build into a swimming program. You will be amazed at how quickly you can increase your water endurance each time. Keep your swimming strokes long and stretched and enjoy your individual progress. Rushing yourself at first will only lead to muscle soreness because your body is not yet used to the exercise.

GETTING BETTER

1. Becoming a better swimmer involves the three basic parts of training known by the abbreviation F.I.T.:

Frequency: One day a week is better than none. Three times a week is recommended for a training effect.
Intensity: Begin at your level, and go slowly. As your skill improves, monitor your heart rate by counting the pulses for fifteen seconds, then multiply by four. If you want to improve your fitness level, you should at least be swimming fast enough to get your heart rate up to 120.
Time: You can begin with as little as ten minutes. To make significant improvements you should train for thirty to sixty minutes.

2. Add variety to your workouts. Try spicing up your distance (continuous) workouts with interval swimming (swimming and resting patterns), kicking with sideboards, pulling with pull-buoys, or a combination of all of these. Motivation and innovation within your program are limited only by your own creativeness.

3. Try working out with a group. Master's Swimming is available throughout the nation, with competition available in five-year age groups. Whatever your level of swimming, remember to swim for the fun of it.

As you become physically active, some other things you may want to consider are the levels of stress in your life and how stress can affect you. You may also be interested in some psychological techniques that can enhance your physical activity. We'll even give you some tips for having a peak performance!

STRESS

We all live with stress in varying degrees and forms. Our bodies are designed to live with a certain amount of stress that is necessary for survival. Eons ago, it was the stress response that allowed humans to run for the hills when a saber-toothed tiger started to stalk them. Today's demands are different, but the body still tries to protect itself, exhibiting behaviors that can take the form of shivering with the cold, or intense anger and fear.

Although a lifestyle with minimal stress sounds ideal, our lives would be very dull without any stress. There are some very positive aspects of stress, among them:

- *Challenge.* We all need a certain amount of challenge in our lives, whether it is in the form of giving a speech, swimming in a timed event, or receiving a hard-earned promotion. It is the challenges that we encounter that keep us stimulated.
- *Change.* Although change can be a very strong stressor, it allows us to grow. With every challenge or change, we become stronger individuals and are more able to cope with later changes.
- *Variety.* A variety of life situations and challenges is the essence of living to your full potential. Without variety our lives become dull and boring.

When a person experiences stress, the nervous and endocrine systems are activated, producing the "fight or flight," or the alarm response. These responses are meant to deal with short-term situations (like getting away from the saber-tooth). Over the long term, the body's physiology becomes altered by these continually overstimulated and activated organs, causing the organs to wear down or become diseased. Stress can also interfere with the normal functioning of the immune system. It is believed that lowered immunity from stress is a major cause of colds, infection, and even cancer. Thus, ironically, the same responses that were intended to facilitate our survival can make us ill if we experience them over a long period of time.

Some other stress-related diseases and disorders include:

Hypertension
Low back pain
Heart disease
Asthma
Duodenal ulcer
Insomnia
Headache

SOURCES OF STRESS

In our day-to-day lives, there are many sources of stress. We don't always have the ability to control or change what is stressful to us. However, simply being aware that something is causing us stress can be a first step to controlling how it will affect us.

Although we may not realize it, our environment can be a source of stress or illness. Loud noise, for instance, can be more than annoying; noise can cause loss of sleep, irritability, permanent hearing loss, and other negative physiological changes. Toxins, carcinogens, and other pollutants in our food and water can slowly but surely be eroding our health. Even the air we depend on can contain substances that cause headaches, sore throats, or even permanent lung problems.

Emotions can also affect our physical health. The negative emotions that can arise in a given day—anxiety, anger, guilt, or frustration—are often natural responses to situations we feel we can't control. Even when circumstances are beyond our control, we may be able to avoid these stress emotions simply by setting some limits. For example, how many times would you have been able to lower your anxiety or frustration level by simply saying, "No, I don't want to do that" or "I'm sorry, I'm too busy"? Yet, for one reason or another, we feel we are unable to do so, putting ourselves in the stressful position of having to do something that we really don't want to do.

The social dimension of our lives is a major contributor to our stress level. Although our relationships with mates, friends, family, and co-workers can be a source of comfort, they can sometimes go awry, causing us a great deal of distress. A change in our economic status, because of the loss of a job or the start of a new career, can shake our foundations to the core. Work is another social stressor for obvious reasons. Not only do we spend a major portion of our lives at work but we also have to perform well, deal with co-workers and bosses, and fit into an organizational culture that may be foreign to us.

Stressors in our personal environment encompass all of the above topics. Our personal environment is everything that surrounds us and affects us or our personal space. This space can be our home or room, our work space, who we live with, how we live, or even what clothes we wear.

Much of our personal space has been arranged by us, so we do have quite a bit of control over it. This control is never complete, however. For example, if we value neatness, we can keep our desk at work tidy, our car clean, and our house picked up. But that works only until our boss throws a pile of work on our desk, the dog has an accident in the car, or our housemate decides to have a party!

Our lifestyle is also part of this personal environment, including the choices and changes that we make. These changes in our lives are perhaps the single greatest source of stress, because they take so much time and energy for us to adapt to them. Often, we compound our stress level by making several major lifestyle changes in a relatively short period of time.

COPING MECHANISMS

Changing Your Perception of the Situation. Our perception of stressful events greatly affects the impact of that event. For example, if we view being laid off from work as a major disaster, our stress level will be high. However, if we see being laid off as a chance for a career change, or the challenge for a better, more satisfying job, our stress level will be much lower.

It is not only how we view an event that determines our level of stress but also how much control we feel we have over our lives. This "locus of control" encompasses several factors, including self-responsible versus victim, luck versus opportunity, and skill versus chance, or internal factors versus external factors. For example, a person believing that external factors control her life may believe that she was hired for her job through luck. A person believing that internal factors control her life may believe that she was hired by having the right skills and convincing the interviewer to hire her.

Generally, our levels of stress are much higher in a situation where we feel that we have no control. Therefore, it can help to realize that we do have some choices in every stressful situation:

- If possible, we can change the situation.
- We can change our reaction to a situation.
- We can change our perception of a situation.

For example, Sara has just been fired from her job. She tries to convince her boss not to fire her. When that fails, she goes home, spends fifteen minutes doing relaxation exercises, and feels better able to handle the situation. She works on changing her perception over the next few days. When she looks at the situation objectively, she is able to admit that she was stagnating in her old job, and that being forced to look for more satisfying employment could be a blessing in disguise.

Exercise. A healthy, well-conditioned body is at the foundation of all stress-coping strategies. For this reason, may people use exercise as their primary source of stress reduction. There are several reasons why exercise works so well. First, vigorous physical activity is a natural outlet for your body when it is in the "fight or flight" stage of arousal. Exercise allows you to work off that adrenaline rush, and afterward, it allows your body to return to its prestress state of equilibrium.

Exercise also allows for periods of relaxed concentration, similar to meditation. This transcendent experience has been called a "runner's high," but can occur in any form of physical activity. It is also believed that endorphins, or pain-killing chemicals released in the brain, are partly responsible for the runner's high. Another benefit of physical activity is the recreation factor, or simply taking the time out from a busy day to enjoy a pleasurable activity.

Nutrition. Even though most of us don't think of proper nutrition as a stress-reduction technique, there are ways that we compound our stress through poor nutrition. An obvious example is high caffeine intake. Caffeine, a stimulant found in coffee, black tea, colas, and chocolate, chemically induces a "fight or flight" response in your body. Therefore, if you are feeling stressed during the day, caffeine will only make matters worse.

Sugar can also affect how you feel. When you eat foods high in sugar, your blood sugar level shoots up, giving you a boost of energy for a short period of time. However, your pancreas produces insulin to counter the sugar in your blood, depressing your blood sugar level to a point lower than before. This low blood sugar can cause dizziness, irritability, depression, shaking, nausea, and hunger pangs that may prompt you to have another sweet snack.

Some people drink alcohol as a form of stress reduction. However, alcohol is a depressant that slows certain functions in some parts of the brain. Alcohol can also irritate the gastrointestinal tract, cause a hangover, and inhibit sleep.

Some nutrition suggestions for lowering stress levels are:

- Eat a good breakfast. A sugary pastry and a cup of coffee do not meet your body's needs for a good breakfast.
- Eat foods high in B vitamins and calcium. If you are under a lot of stress, these nutrients will be even more important.
- Eat a wide variety of foods to ensure that you are getting enough nutrients.
- Eat four or five small meals a day. Frequent eating avoids stress associated with hunger and keeps blood sugar even.
- Take the time to eat. Eat slowly and enjoy the relaxation that comes from eating good food in unharried surroundings.

Relationships. The relationships in your life can be a real godsend when you are feeling particularly stressed. Sometimes, coming home and sharing the highlights of a particularly trying day with your partner can be the most effective way of diffusing stress. Also, recreational time spent with family can be very relaxing.

Close friends can support you by listening or offering another perspective in a problem situation. Individual counseling or support groups can also be good places to air your anxieties and reduce your stress. Depending on where you live, you can often find support groups that focus on almost any topic, be it men's or women's issues, work, uncoupling, chemical dependency, or even exercise addiction!

Relaxation Techniques. Relaxation techniques can be very effective in dealing with stress. There are many forms of relaxation techniques, including biofeedback, meditation, self-hypnosis, visualization, guided imagery, and progressive relaxation. Many of these techniques are covered in the sports psychology section of this chapter.

Massage is also an effective form of stress reduction. Massage can be both relaxing and energizing, providing increased circulation, relief from tension headaches and backaches, and faster healing of muscle strains and injuries.

Other effective ways of receiving stress are Eastern practices such as acupressure or acupuncture. Acupressure or acupuncture is the opening and balancing of energy through relaxation or stimulation of various pressure points of the body. T'ai chi, a form of soft exercise, incorporates slow, simple movement with relaxation. By practicing this ancient form of Chinese exercise, you can improve balance, flexibility, and breathing, while achieving a calmness of body and mind. For many, the practice of yoga is considered to be the ultimate in stress reduction. Yoga involves a series of postures that cause a slow, passive stretching of the muscles, promoting the free flow of energy and relaxation.

Whatever form of relaxation you choose, it is important to practice it on a regular basis for effective results. An added benefit of practicing stress reduction exercises is the fact that you will be spending quiet time alone, allowing you a reprieve from your busy day.

SPORT PSYCHOLOGY

Once you have been involved with an activity for a while, you may reach a plateau where you aren't seeing any improvement. A variety of factors, including stress or some sort of mental block, may be keeping you from doing your best. Some athletes have found that certain mental exercises help them get past the plateau stage so their performance can begin to improve again.

Sport psychology is a relatively new discipline that applies the concepts of psychology to the area of athletics. Like any scientific endeavor, it attempts to observe, describe, explain, predict, and ultimately control the behavior of an athlete in order to improve performance. The applications range from learning how to deal with a losing season to improving a skill through mental imagery. Here are some sport psychology techniques that you may want to explore on your own to help you improve in any activity, be it athletic or not.

Progressive Relaxation. We all worry and are anxious about our performance from time to time, whether it is an upcoming competition or a big job interview. Some amount of anxiety is expected, and can actually increase performance, but too much of it can prevent you from doing your best. When you are too tense to think clearly or to concentrate, your performance is bound to suffer. The ability to relax "on call" can be helpful.

Progressive relaxation is called progressive because different muscle groups are alternately contracted and relaxed during the learning process. For example, start with your toes, tightening them as tight as you can, then relaxing them, taking time to feel the difference. Next, go to your calves and repeat the procedure, working your way up your body until even your forehead and scalp are relaxed. Eventually, you can relax just by thinking about it, almost anytime and anywhere.

Goal Setting. Quite simply, setting a goal means identifying what you want to accomplish and why you want to accomplish it. Goals can range from walking around the block without resting to winning a gold medal in the Olympics. They should be realistic, measurable, and related to performance, but most of all, they should be challenging enough to motivate you. Goals are effective only when they are truly important to you. Because each person is motivated differently, only you can set your own goals.

Self-talk. Repeating positive messages to yourself before a competition or important event can enhance and reinforce your self-confidence and positive mental attitude. It can provide a sense of control and awareness about your feelings, which creates a self-fulfilling prophecy. The first step is to be aware of what you are currently saying to yourself. If you hear yourself saying, "I am afraid I am not going to perform well," you can check this negative thought and turn it into, "I am nervous, but I will perform well."

Imagery/Mental Practice. This process involves going through an experience in your mind and practicing it, using thought and imagination. It is most effective when you evoke vivid, realistic images that contain information like smell, sight, sound, taste, and feeling. Studies have shown that this tool is very effective to use along with physical practice to improve performance. You can either feel what it is like to go through an activity step by step, or you can imagine that you are a spectator, watching yourself perform the activity. For example, a swimmer might go through the race in her head, from the time she is standing on the starting block to the time she touches the finish. Since the goal in imagery is to improve performance, she can even make herself the winner. She can experience the feelings of her muscles stretching and pulling, her increase in breathing, and the thoughts that run through her head. She can even use self-talk as she goes. In the next scenario, she can watch herself cross the finish line, and even see the race clock displaying the time that she would like to achieve. However, in order for the practice to be effective in improving performance, the action must be performed correctly. Like physical practice, if you practice it using the wrong technique or form, it can be counterproductive.

Hypnosis/Self-hypnosis. This technique has become quite popular in athletic circles lately. During hypnosis, you achieve a deep state of mental and physical relaxation in which your mind is open to suggestions. In this way, hypnosis incorporates pieces of relaxation, mental imagery, and even self-talk. It can help a person overcome inhibitions and increase confidence, but it does not create attributes that the person does not already have. For instance, hypnosis can help athletes express existing strengths that they have been unable or unwilling to express before, but it cannot create new strengths. This technique is limited, however, because only about 30 percent of the population can reach an effective state of hypnosis. It is also important to check on the qualifications and experience of the hypnotist.

Systematic Desensitization. This technique can help you reduce your fear of a specific situation by using progressive muscle relaxation techniques. After first being taught to master relaxation, you are then subjected to a series of progressively more fearful situations and taught to relax during them. By reducing anxiety, relaxation also reduces the fear during these simulated situations. Eventually, you can learn to apply the technique to a real situation. For example, a pitcher on a softball team who throws well during practice but poorly during games would be taught to relax during gamelike situations. Eventually, she would be able to apply what she has learned to shed her fear during real games.

Attentional Focus. Research shows that mistakes often occur when our attention is focused on the wrong thing. There are many kinds of attention, and we switch between them freely during the day. Internal attention is focused on the thoughts and feelings of the self, whereas external attention is focused on the environment surrounding the self. Narrow attention is focused on only one thing, whereas broad attention is directed at many different things. We use different kinds of attention depending on the task. Writing a paper, for instance, requires internal, narrow attention to gather thoughts and transfer them to the paper. When driving a car, we need broad, external attention to focus on what other drivers are doing, on road signs, and on where we are going. You can improve your concentration in many areas by simply learning to recognize what type of focus you are using, and then changing it to suit your needs.

Some of these techniques, such as hypnosis, require the help of another person. At the present time, there are no regulations or standards for the designation of sport psychologist. To find a sports oriented psychologist, you may want to seek referrals from the local chapter of the American Psychological Association or from other people who have worked with someone they trust. Once you find a practitioner, make an appointment just to ask questions and get a feel for whether you can work with this person. You should feel comfortable and relaxed and be able to trust his or her judgment and advice. Make sure whoever you work with is willing to refer you to someone else if necessary.

PEAK PERFORMANCE

Have you ever experienced a peak performance in your athletic activity? At Melpomene, we were curious to find out what our members had to say about peak performances. Were they something that only elite athletes experienced? Was a peak performance the same as a "runner's high"? Did it only happen to runners, or could cyclists, swimmers, and golfers experience the same thing? Would peak performances only happen in structured, competitive situations?

Our members responded enthusiastically to our survey. Some considered peak performance to be the same as *peak experience*—a term that was originally coined by Abraham Maslow, the humanistic psychologist. Maslow believed that a self-actualized person could expect to have peak experiences—moments of highest happiness and fulfillment, characterized by loss of fears, inhibitions, and insecurities. These moments were of total peace and well-being. This definition refers to a subjective emotional state.

Other Melpomene members saw peak performance in terms of objective measures of success, such as when they had won a race or achieved a personal best. This view of peak performance is common among many people in sports, especially those in competitive sports. Of course, the subjective feeling that Maslow talks about may occur at the same time the objective record is being broken. What our Melpomene members taught us is that there need not be a medal or a trophy at the end of the race in order to experience a peak performance. All that's really needed is a sense of accomplishment.

For example, one woman wrote, "I ran my first marathon . . . and the emotional and physical high . . . can only compare to childbirth." Another woman recalled that after her first marathon, "I cried I was so happy. Never had I felt such a sense of accomplishment. I had done something totally on my own and succeeded."

Peak performances seem to be characterized by (1) relaxation, (2) a sense of power and energy, (3) a feeling of being focused and in control, and (4) an experience of joy and freedom. Quotes from members participating in many different activities reveal these characteristics. It is also clear that a peak performance is a very personal, self-defined accomplishment.

"When I ran my first twenty-mile race . . . I had an overwhelming sense of my body as a finely tuned piece of machinery, and I had control over all the gears. I was able to shift gears for hills and visualized my hips as if the gears were similar to those on my bike. It was an amazing experience to me and the feeling that I had complete control of my performance turned out to be very relaxing."

"In 1980, my whole ski season was incredible. Every race was good— I was fast and felt terrific. The last race was great—felt in control and on top of things the whole way—a fantastic experience!"

"During the finals of the national singles championship in 1971, the background blended together and I was aware of nothing but the shuttlecock. I was totally oblivious to fatigue and pain, and my movements felt smooth and gliding, without conscious effort."

"In long-distance canoe races I feel very in touch with self and environment—a wonderful sense of mastery and accomplishment."

THE BARRIERS TO PEAK PERFORMANCE

The joy that physical activity brings is too great to be restricted to just one-half of the population. And yet, for a variety of social and psychological reasons, women do not have the same opportunity as men to participate and develop their skills in physical activity and sport. Without the chance to participate and grow, many women live their whole lives without experiencing a peak performance through physical activity.

Our concept of sex roles is one barrier that has kept women from achieving their peak performance. At least three different models for sex role stereotyping have been proposed: bipolar, androgynous, and transcendent. According to the bipolar model, sex roles are composed of two mutually exclusive clusters of characteristics. Men have their trademark characteristics, women have theirs, and the two never overlap.

People who believe in the bipolar model see an athletic woman as a contradiction in terms. This kind of thinking forces a woman into a classic double-bind situation: If I am an athlete I cannot be a woman. If I am a woman I cannot be an athlete. How is a female athlete supposed to cope with the perception that her two identities are mutually exclusive? She has several choices, including dropping out of sports, devaluing her athletic abilities, pursuing only "acceptable" sports (i.e., those that call for traditionally feminine characteristics such as grace), or engaging in what sport sociologist Susan Birrell calls "apologetic" behaviors. An example of apologetic behavior is when a woman makes a point of wearing jewelry and makeup while playing sports so as to prove her femininity.

Obviously, this kind of role conflict can erode our athletic performance if we allow it to have power over us. Instead, we might adopt the androgynous sex role model that says men and women do not have discreet and exclusive sets of characteristics. Androgynous people possess a range of both feminine and masculine characteristics, and the traits that they display depend on circumstances. In the androgynous model, women are not faced with a role conflict when they engage in physical activity or sport. They don't need to devalue or deny their so-called female traits such as expressiveness, and they can acknowledge and develop those traits that are deemed more male, such as an interest in athletics.

The third sex role model—the transcendent model—does not focus on sex roles or masculine versus feminine at all. Perhaps someday we can go beyond such labels and have this kind of gender-free model that will encourage everyone to maximize their potential in whatever area they choose. To see where our physically active respondents stood on sex role modeling, we looked carefully at the way they described themselves. More than 50 percent of the women characterized themselves as nurturing, successful, happy, sensitive, versatile, and friendly. These traits are all in keeping with the feminine role. On the other hand, the majority also believed themselves to be athletic, competitive, and independent—all masculine traits. Happily, few felt that social disapproval in the form of ridicule, lack of encouragement, or social pressure was an obstacle to being physically active. The only major obstacle these women cited was the lack of time to exercise given the demands put on them by jobs and family. We see this obstacle as an indirect effect of sex role modeling on athletic women, however. It seems that most of society still expects women to do double duty: raising kids and running a household while also holding down a job outside the home.

Another limitation to peak performance is the way many women view achievement. Because women have only just begun to be accepted in high-stakes athletics, we are still not used to seeing women accomplish great physical feats, which makes it hard for many of us to take ourselves seriously in the realm of sports. A woman who has low expectations about her own ability to perform is quick to attribute her success to luck rather than to ability. Think about how difficult it would be to motivate yourself in practice if you honestly believed, as many women do, that your performance hinges on luck rather than on skill!

PEAK PERFORMANCE FROM A WOMAN'S POINT OF VIEW

Women also seem to differ from men in the reasons they give for participating in sport. Although 75 percent of the respondents in our membership survey compete in their sport, only one-third said that the chance to test themselves, to succeed or fail, was a very significant part of being physically active. In fact, 70 percent stated that the chance to compete is not at all important to them. For these women, achievement in sport is not necessarily measured by how well they do compared to an externally imposed standard. It may be that internal or intrinsic rewards such as greater self-esteem are the prime motivators for women, even in competitive events.

This view may not be the traditionally "masculine" way to view sports, but is there anything wrong with it? Actually, there are a lot of benefits associated with performing for personal rather than for public glory. When internal motivators are at the helm, sports become satisfying whether there are external rewards or not. That satisfaction is no longer reserved for a select few. For instance, the older athlete, who cannot hope to "win" against the younger athlete, can still enjoy the race. Also, for people who are actually distracted by external rewards, internal rewards may inspire peak performances.

The only danger we can see in internal motivators is if women set their sights too high or too low. How we set our standards is in many ways a result of how we were raised. When asked about sources of support for their physical activity, our respondents mentioned family, peers, and other socializing agents, like schools. And, of course, sex role stereotyping can also come from all of these sources. As Billie Jean King has observed, "It all starts with pink and blue blankets." A more extensive discussion of sport socialization, and Melpomene's research in this area can be found beginning on page 148.

Younger women have been raised in an era when the androgynous sex role model was more accepted. Androgyny, though an improvement over the pink-and-blue-blanket syndrome, still implies a deficit model for women in sports. Women are advised to develop their instrumental, masculine traits in order to fully participate in the male-dominated sporting arena, and are in effect told to leave their feminine characteristics at home. Don't women have something valuable to offer? We believe that the expressive, cooperative, and participatory emphasis of women might be a healthy counter to the often destructive "winning is everything" ethic frequently found in sport.

Hopefully, we will someday reach that transcendent, gender-free status in which behavior is appropriate not because it is feminine or masculine but because it fits the situation. In sport, whatever we must do to reach the peaks of individual potential is appropriate. Peak performances occur when two simple factors meet—challenge and ability. If we remove the barriers that keep girls and women from fully participating in sport, we can in time raise our levels of both challenge and ability. In this way more of us will be able to experience peak performance, and the peaks to which we aspire will be higher.

One reason for thinking about peak performance is not just to push athletes higher, farther, and faster but to return to the basic motivation for sport—the sheer joy and pleasure of using our bodies. When asked, "What is the best part of physical activity?" one of our members succinctly stated, "It's feeling *great* instead of just good." To strive for that experience through physical activity is a wonderful way to take care of yourself.

E I G H T

CONVERSATIONS WITH NINE ACTIVE WOMEN

There's nothing more inspiring than seeing a woman's eyes light up when she talks about her favorite activity. We had that experience when we interviewed nine women, ages twenty-four to eighty-two, for this chapter. These women all had decided to make regular exercise a vital part of their lives. They were vibrant with enthusiasm for their active lifestyles, but they also told us about the parts of exercise that were hard for them. We got a true-to-life picture of how women of different ages, backgrounds, and skill levels get involved in physical activity, and how they stay involved throughout the various stages of their lives. In this final chapter, we'd like to share their stories with you, in hopes that you can see a part of yourself in their spirit.

To give context to the interviews and provide you with background information to relate to your specific situation, we began by asking about preferred physical activity. Because the women selected are different ages, we thought it was important to know about their experiences as a child and teenager. We also knew you would be interested in how each woman got started, how often they do their physical activity, and how important it was to receive encouragement. We also asked about exercise and relationships, injuries, and how being physically active changed food preferences and general dietary practices. Finally we asked each woman how she "takes care of herself."

HARRIET, age eighty-two

"At my age, swimming is my favorite and best activity," says Harriet. She has just returned from a trip to Africa that included a safari, ballooning, and a rough, bone-shaking jeep ride. Harriet says the jeep ride aggravated her back problem, but even so, she wouldn't have missed it for the world. People who first meet Harriet are amazed by her stamina and love of life, but those who know her well say that Harriet has always thrived on activity, adventure, and learning new things.

When we asked her what she liked to do as a young child, her response was simple: "I liked everything!" As a teenager she loved tennis, horseback riding, canoeing, and camping. She recalls that although there were few organized sports for women in those days, the local YWCA did have a team that competed against several other teams in the area. In high school, she participated in AAU swimming, which was one of the few sports open to women. In college, Harriet managed to get an athletic letter by participating in almost every intermural sport available. By the time she was a junior, she decided to switch her major from medical technology to physical education. "In addition to just loving all the sports, I started thinking about my own free time," she says. "I figured if I became a lab tech I would have three weeks of vacation, but as a teacher I would have the whole summer free to travel." In her six years as a physical educator, she became more versatile and experienced in various sports, but swimming remained her favorite.

Harriet can't recall any time when she wasn't physically active. After she quit teaching high school, she taught swimming. Harriet helped design and construct one of the first private outdoor pools in her city and gave formal and informal lessons to hundreds of kids and adults over the years.

Swimming is still her favorite activity. Because she is not an early riser, she frequently swims at eleven or twelve in the morning, after enjoying a leisurely breakfast, reading the paper, or planning another trip. In the early afternoon, she's usually out somewhere, volunteering, exploring, or visiting friends. On days when she misses her swim in the morning, she tries to work it in before coming home for dinner.

Harriet did not have a lot of encouragement to be active as a child, but she doesn't recall any discouragement either. "Mostly," she says, "my parents and others didn't seem to care one way or the other." Today she says most of her contemporaries aren't into athletics at all. She therefore seeks out friends, particularly young people, who are also active. She contributes time and dollars to provide college scholarships for women athletes. Realizing how much she herself has gained, and sorry that more opportunities did not exist when she was young, Harriet wants to be sure that young women have more chances for continued improvement in their sport. She thinks that being involved with sports at an early age can benefit a woman well into the later years of her life.

As she has gotten older, Harriet has had to adjust to the bodily changes that come with a full life. A car accident fifty years ago, resulting in a fractured knee, curtailed her downhill skiing. Other than that, she feels lucky to have been able to do most anything she wanted throughout most of her life. Harriet admits that aches and pains have begun to slow her down in recent years, but she is actively working to alleviate problems so that "it is more fun to go on long walks again." She tells us with a grin that she still challenges anyone half her age to try and keep up with her.

Harriet has also changed food preferences and habits over the years. She doesn't eat sweets or chocolates, mostly because she wants to keep her weight down. She also follows a low-salt and low-fat diet and eats little meat. She says she has always loved milk and continues to drink it on a daily basis. "I don't have to worry about my calcium intake!"

Activity "absolutely" changes the way Harriet perceives her body. "Knowing that I am physically capable gives me great confidence. Even though it may be harder to get started these days, I know that physical activity will make me feel better. So I do it!" Harriet believes taking care of yourself is very important. For Harriet this means regular medical checkups. Two cancer surgeries, both many years ago, have kept her tuned in to her body. She makes sure that she eats regularly and closely monitors her medications.

Harriet says one of the best ways for her to take care of herself is to continually seek new knowledge and new experiences. At age twenty-two she spent two months on a ship in the Middle East, at a time when women did not travel alone. Since that time she has traveled around the world, finding new friends and sharing her adventures when she returns. Being adventuresome and physically active makes life rich and fun!

NANCY, age twenty-four

Nancy likes running, swimming, biking, and hiking. When she was a child, she had a love/hate relationship with swimming, but her fascination with water polo could keep her in the water for hours. She picked up water polo from her family and friends, and was fortunate to be able to compete on a team in high school. Nancy realizes that she has had many more choices and opportunities connected with sport than women who are older.

Besides being born in an era when girl's athletics were getting more support, Nancy was also born into a family that always seemed to be doing something that was physically active and fun. Her family's lifestyle made it easier, she thinks, to be with friends who also liked to do similar things. As a result, Nancy reports that she doesn't think there has ever been a period of time when she wasn't physically active—"Well, except for a couple of days during exam week!"

As she was growing up, being physically active helped Nancy define who she was. In high school, she competed in water polo and swimming, and in college she joined the cross-country running team. "I have never been a star athlete or seen competition as particularly important," she says. "I was competitive enough to make the team, but was never outstanding." The best part of being on a team was the chance to share her activity with others, and the experience convinced her that physical activity of some sort would always play a part in her life.

Today, several years out of college, Nancy finds that running can be either a social or an individual pursuit. She loves, for instance, the time she spends running with her Hash group. Hash groups were begun by British diplomats who had appointments in foreign countries. The purpose of the exercise is to catch the lead group of runners who are following a devious route. It's a social sort of competition that encourages people of all abilities. On her own, Nancy tries to do something physical every day and frequently chooses to run because it is so convenient. Her second choice is to go for a hike. Because she has never tried a triathlon before and thinks it would be fun, she is swimming and riding her bike more frequently.

Nancy prefers to exercise in the late afternoon or evening, although she says that a lot of factors, including how much time is available, figure into her daily decision on when to work out. She credits self-motivation and her lifelong pattern of exercise for making it easy to fit physical activity into her day. She says that although she was never discouraged by outside forces, she has always found that most of her encouragement comes from inside. "Intellectually and emotionally, I know it's important for me to exercise every day."

Nancy says that she doesn't compete often enough to let an upcoming race alter her eating or sleeping patterns, but remembers a time when she did.

> In high school and college, I was more compulsive about eating the "right things," and more rigid about not letting myself gain weight. I would never allow myself anything made with butter or any sweets, for instance. I used to think being thinner would make me a better runner, but I don't think that's true anymore. It's not that I've drastically changed my eating habits in the past three or four years. I guess the best way to describe it is to say that I am more relaxed. I enjoy a lot of foods and have drifted back to freer, less restricted eating.

Nancy thinks being physically active definitely influences the way she sees her body. She thinks her changing perception of the importance of being thin is a very positive change. She feels strong, competent, and able to do almost anything she would like to do physically.

Nancy has already learned that a hectic work schedule can sometimes get in the way of taking care of herself. Her most recent job involved working on a fund-raising effort where she finally limited herself to a twelve-hour working day. "That left time to come home, run, and sleep." She laughs ruefully. "I quickly learned that I don't want to work even a nine-hour day, but sometimes dedication to the job makes it easy for that to happen." Nancy says she also realized that she didn't like to spend that much time in one place; she's decided to look for more flexibility as well as shorter hours in her next job.

Nancy has always learned that being creative gives her a lot of energy. This spring, for fun, she took a course in short-story writing, and surprisingly found that she had a talent for writing poetry! The writing proved to be a wonderful form of therapy, and Nancy vowed that she would make more time to do her own writing. She also started looking for jobs that would allow her to use her writing skills more often. For Nancy, taking care of herself means nurturing both the athletic and the creative parts of her personality. It means balancing her life to include time for working out, time for being with friends, and time to be alone so she can think and write.

WENDY, age thirty-four

Wendy is probably the most serious athlete of the group interviewed for this chapter. As a member of a national basketball team, she has access to coaches, as well as expert information about diet and sleep. She works out four or five times a week, and when she is not competing in basketball, archery, or road racing, she has a job helping other people become physically active. The feature that really sets Wendy apart, however, is that she experiences all her victories while using a wheelchair.

Before she was disabled, Wendy enjoyed swimming and playing pick-up games of kickball and softball. There was little else for girls to do in her small hometown because the only organized sports teams were for boys. When she was fourteen, Wendy injured her spinal cord in a car accident, and her days in the pool and playground came to a halt. No one knew much about kids in wheelchairs in her small town, and no one even thought about involving Wendy in sports. Luckily, her high school was relatively new and all on one floor, so she was at least able to continue her classes.

The four years following her accident were difficult because Wendy had no role models and little self-confidence. She gained weight, and because she thought disabled people couldn't participate in sports, she never considered working out as a way to slim down. When it came time for college, her parents urged her to apply; they themselves had never had the opportunity for higher education and were convinced that it could open doors for Wendy.

Wendy chose a school that had an excellent program for disabled students. Suddenly, after four years of having no peers in her situation, she met other people using wheelchairs. To her surprise, many of them were physically active, and they encouraged her to join them. At first, it took quite a lot of persuading. One graduate assistant who also served as a coach for disabled athletes played a major role in convincing Wendy to give it a try. Because she had been coordinated as a child, Wendy found that this natural ability showed itself quickly. "I found I was good at many of the activities, and of course this encouraged me to continue." By the end of her first year of college, Wendy decided to join an archery team and compete. The combination of being more physically active, enjoying competition, and developing a more positive body image also helped Wendy lose the weight she had gained in high school.

Eventually, Wendy decided that she would like a career helping other people enjoy physical activity. She earned a master's degree in leisure studies and got a job as a therapeutic recreation specialist at a rehabilitation and treatment center for people with disabilities. These days, she usually fits her physical activity into the end of her workday or on weekends.

Wendy feels she is lucky to live in a community where there are many opportunities for disabled athletes. She belongs to a basketball team that practices regularly and has an active season against other teams. In the summer she can find a road race to enter almost every weekend, and there are numerous archery competitions. On the national front, she was a member of the 1988 Paralympics basketball team that competed in Seoul, Korea. Wendy would encourage other women with disabilities to seriously consider these opportunities and possibilities when making career or educational decisions. Wendy finds that the friends she has made through her physical activities are an extremely important part of her positive outlook on life.

Once people get over their stereotypes about what someone who uses a wheelchair can do, they are usually supportive. One of the problems young children with disabilities face, however, is the fear parents and others have about their safety. Because Wendy remembers how lonely it was to be without role models as a teenager, she frequently volunteers to help kids realize that their disability does not prohibit them from trying all kinds of sports. Wendy lists a great variety of physical activities including golf and tennis as things she likes to do recreationally.

Through both her competitive and recreational pursuits, Wendy has experienced several overuse injuries, including tendonitis of the elbow and wrist. She also broke two fingers. Her worst injury only kept her out of action for three weeks, however. Now she is more careful and can usually predict when she is getting close to an injury. Since she works just down the hall from the latest sports medicine equipment, she can also get minor therapy quickly and easily.

Wendy says she can never forget to take care of herself. She says that ignoring the fact that she has a spinal cord injury would be "stupid." Because the accident left her with no sensation, she must be particularly careful of the air temperature and what happens to her skin. Any major problem could be disruptive not only for competition but for her job and other activities. So far, Wendy has experienced few interruptions related to her physical self. "I'm careful not to let myself get too tired, and to take time off when I become aware of changes in my body." Wendy also knows that she needs personal time to "regroup," so she always schedules time to read and play the piano.

Physical activity has obviously played a pivotal part in Wendy's life. Through participation in sport she was able to change her self-image and body image, gain recognition as an athlete, and discover that she wanted to be professionally involved in this area. Many of her friends are people who she has met through competition and who share her ambitions and dreams. When asked how she sees her future, Wendy says, "I would like to compete for many more years because it is so much fun, but even if I'm not competing, I know that I'll be physically active for the rest of my life."

PEG, age fifty-one

Peg's favorite physical activities are walking and orienteering. She has also taken a variety of exercise classes regularly over the past twenty-five years. Wherever she lives (and she's moved around a lot), finding an exercise class is one of the first things she does. She does bike, but for her, the bicycle is mainly a means of transportation.

Peg remembers playing ballgames at school because they were compulsory, not because she enjoyed them. She grew up in a rural area where she had to ride her bike to get anywhere, and she recalls these rides as the only physical activity she got during her teenage years. She says that during her twenties she really didn't do anything. "Oh, I did a little fencing because my spouse was doing it, but it was never very important."

Peg, who is British, has lived in the United States and Canada for nearly one-third of her married life. Her favorite sport—orienteering— was begun in England and is still more popular and organized there than it is here. Nevertheless, Peg and her husband found a small group that was meeting sporadically on Sundays and decided to join them. For the first several years, Peg attended meets but says she mostly "walked round with the kids who were very tiny at the time." Orienteering meets are usually held in parks or wooded areas. Before the meet, organizers set numbered markers in the woods and note their location on a map. Participants use a compass and a copy of the map to help them move from point to point. The goal is to find all the markers and complete the course as quickly as possible. Usually several courses are set and individuals choose the one that is appropriate for their ability and age.

Peg found the company at orienteering meets congenial; there were several other young families and the whole day was a nice low-key family outing. Gradually the women began to pool childcare so that those who wanted to could set out on their own without the kids. In much of Europe, orienteering meets are held almost every weekend, but in the United States, it is more likely that they will be held once or twice a month. If the group is dedicated enough, meets are held year-round, even in snowbound Minnesota.

When asked about competition, Peg says that she is not a competitive person and doesn't particularly mind that she rarely "wins" anything. On the few occasions when she has won something in her age category at an orienteering meet, she admits it "pleases her," but also thinks her two sons and spouse are more excited than she is. Peg also points out that orienteering is a unique sport. "It is an intellectual as well as physical exercise. Frequently the winner is not the fastest runner, but the person who cleverly figures out the cues and miscues. I have a great sense of achievement when I have completed a difficult course without making a mistake!"

The only way one might practice orienteering is to also be a runner, an activity that holds little interest for Peg. She much prefers to walk, usually in the mid- to late morning. "I'm absolutely hopeless the first thing in the morning! If it doesn't fit my schedule at that time I'm likely to wait until late afternoon."

When asked about encouragement, Peg says that her parents knew she disliked games and therefore didn't push her to participate. She says her spouse is always "nagging" her to be active. (Nagging does not translate directly, it is more a sense of encouragement as used by the British!) She thinks that her family's encouragement helps her to be more regular about exercise.

Peg has probably tried more exercise classes than anyone else interviewed. She says she really tries to find one all the time. It has been a quick way to make some new connections as she has traveled around the world. Peg isn't particular about the kind of class and has tried yoga, aerobics, stretching, and free weights. The most important criterion in choosing a class is to find a good instructor and Peg feels that she has become skilled in making that judgment over the years. "I've been very pleased with community education classes, but I do ask the instructor about qualifications and then carefully observe the way the class is conducted."

Peg says that she has changed food preferences and habits over the years but doesn't relate that to physical activity. Her diet has become healthier as she has moved toward more fruits, vegetables, and less sweets. "Of course," she says laughing, "one of my favorite activities is to cook really good meals for friends, and then I don't always prepare things that are so healthy!"

While Peg does not consider physical activity a major factor in her feeling of well-being and self-care, she also says that she could never be a couch potato. She knows that taking exercise classes makes her look and feel better. She particularly likes the feeling that she is more flexible and that exercise means that she can eliminate "odd bits of flab."

Peg sees herself as a people-oriented woman who seeks out new acquaintances and likes to be involved with people on a daily basis. Yet she also treasures time alone and can bury herself in a book quite happily. Because her husband travels a lot and her children are grown, she feels that her ability to make friends and be content with her own company enhances her feeling of well-being.

EMILY, age seventy-four

Emily takes a walk every day, and at least five times a week she completes the three-mile circuit around a lake near her home. By preference she walks early in the morning when both she and the day are at their best! She might swim more, she says, if there was a pool nearby. When she's visiting her daughter in Florida, for instance, she swims daily.

Emily couldn't remember any particular sports activity that she focused on as a child. "I lived in a small town, we ran around a lot, and did pick-up sports, fun things, but not something that could really be defined as sport." Emily rode her bike frequently, skated, and played basketball and volleyball when they were offered at school.

Her life has always included some sort of physical activity. When her children were little she swam one day a week and bowled several times per week. Bowling was her regular activity until she went back to school in her early fifties. Studying then became a priority and it became difficult to fit her schedule into league time so she began to walk more and to define that as physical activity.

Emily says that the only time she viewed herself as competitive was when she was bowling regularly. She doesn't recall any particular person encouraging or discouraging her. Except, she says, laughing, " My grandson got a trampoline that I just loved! I would always use it when we visited!" That activity did produce comments and admonitions, especially from her spouse who said she was too old to be engaging in such activity!

Emily definitely feels that exercise affects relationships. "It gives me perspective on things," she says. "I really like to walk alone; it's time akin to prayer or meditation. It gives me a chance to get in touch with the center of me and work off the adrenaline. I find my sense of humor. It's very hard to articulate because it is primarily an emotional thing." Part of the sense of well-being that Edith receives from walking is being outside. In her words, "the world gets bigger, you feel like you're part of the larger universe." By enriching herself in this way, Edith feels that she has more to bring to her relationships.

When we asked about injuries, Emily could only recall one. One day in the midst of her walk, she developed a pain in her foot that grew so bad it kept her on the couch with ice packs for the next four days. "That was long enough to let me know I didn't like being inactive," she remembers. There was a brief period, following a mastectomy at age sixty-five, when she consciously felt a need to exercise her body, particularly her upper torso. Thankfully, the surgery did very little to damage her body image or her sense of well-being. Soon after the surgery Emily distinctly recalls looking in the mirror and thinking, "It don't look all that bad; I look like a Picasso painting." Emily says that her readjustment period was very short, perhaps two or three weeks. "Two things helped me keep my spirits up," she says: "I wasn't thirty and my spouse was wonderful." It is clear to those who see Emily on her walks around the lake that she feels healthy and likes the way she looks. "I have always liked my body," she says, "and I'm very good at self-talk."

Emily claims to have a cast-iron stomach and a wide range of food preferences, but says her food habits have changed over the years. She now "treats" herself to butter on an occasional basis and eats practically no sugar. She has reduced her meat intake to once a week and only has desserts once every two weeks. She has also eliminated the drink before dinner, which she really enjoys but feels isn't good for her weight. "I realize that I have to eat less as I get older," she says. "My metabolism isn't as fast as it once was." The move toward healthier foods was prompted by Emily's reading and her general awareness that these choices would be better for both her and her husband.

Emily is good at listening to her body and taking care of herself. She rises early by choice, is very active during the day, and finds that not letting herself get too tired is important as she gets older. She has found that a short nap can do wonders. She is quick to add that although she rests when she needs to, she refuses to coddle herself or to use her age as an excuse. She feels that too many people speed the aging process by becoming old mentally.

One of the hardest things for Emily is deciding how to divide her time among her many interests. She has always liked being where the action is, yet knows that she needs time alone to recharge herself. "But not too much time," she says. "Feeling isolated or lonesome is bad for me." Emily sees her friends whenever she can, and keeps in close touch with those who no longer live near her through long, interesting letters for which she is famous. Being connected through personal contacts and letters helps her feel "a part of the world." For many years Emily headed a nationally acclaimed educational program for women, and she continues to take classes so that she can stay alive intellectually. "I love my class," she says. "The participants include women of all ages and backgrounds. The two hours I spend there gives me something to think about all week long!"

JEAN, age forty-one

Jean quickly lists several activities as her favorites including running, biking, and cross-country skiing. She also mentions her exercycle but says that being outside comes first, and inside activities are only for "emergencies," like 98-degree heat and humidity or 32 degrees below zero!

Jean remembers very few organized sports activities as a child. She liked to swim and go bike riding but some of her fondest memories include "running around and playing around" with neighborhood friends. "We just had a lot of fun playing kick-the-can, pick-up softball, and hide-and-seek. All of these things seem unsophisticated and almost hard for my daughters to comprehend, but I think that kind of background has had a positive influence on the way I act today."

While she viewed herself as an active child, Jean reports that she did practically nothing during her teenage years. Being physically active was considered somewhat weird by her peers in an all-girl high school. While she found most gym glasses to be unimaginative and boring, one of her physical education teachers served as a role model. Mainly because of this woman, Jean decided to study physical education in college.

Interestingly, Jean describes her college years as being inactive. When questioned she realized that she was taking physical education classes that involved playing and learning to teach every imaginable sport for as many as three hours per day. This variety and experience with sport was required for certification as an elementary P.E. teacher. Yet Jean saw those activities as classes, rather than as participation, and "did nothing" that was physically active outside of her required courses.

She shocked herself into a running program during her first year of teaching. "I was administering the president's physical fitness tests and was appalled at how badly my students were doing. Then one boy who was reasonably good challenged me to try the 400-meter run, and I realized I would have difficulty completing it. I started running soon after!"

For the past twenty years Jean has run, walked, or biked six days per week. She finds weekends are the hardest time to be sure she has time; family plans become important and scheduling sometimes seems impossible. Today, her busy schedule of finishing her Ph.D., parenting, and volunteering encourages her to get up early and meet a group to go running. "I'm always motivated then, and it seems easiest to fit it into my day; if I don't do it then, I waste time scheduling instead of just running."

Jean, who was diagnosed with diabetes twelve years ago, always has to be sure to monitor her food intake before a run. She prides herself on taking care of her body, but is occasionally frustrated when her body reacts in an unusual way. Several weeks ago, for instance, her blood sugar plummeted during a run, and the other runners in her group had to help her home. Despite incidents like these, Jean refuses to let her diabetes control her life, or her love and need for physical activity. One of her goals was to run a marathon, and she was able to do it by carefully regulating her diet. Since then, she's competed in two fifty-two-kilometer cross-country ski races. She is, however, very careful in these circumstances and is constantly searching for new information that will help her better understand her condition. Unfortunately, the formal medical world does not have a great deal of information on physical activity and diabetes. She is pleased that the International Diabetes Center, located in Minneapolis, is starting a society for the study of diabetic athletes.

Although Jean enjoys the comradeship and excitement of an occasional five- or ten-kilometer road race, and was on a swim team for two summers as a child, she says she usually avoids competition. "Being physically active has helped define who I am, but I have never seen myself as an 'athlete.' I run for my own pleasure and well-being." Jean is pleased to tell us about her two daughters who are "potentially excellent athletes" who play soccer and swim. She also notes that their opportunities are different; their schools have encouraged sports for girls and they have had the chance to be on teams with good coaches.

Jean has experienced one major sports-related injury and she is determined it won't happen again. In 1984, a pelvic stress fracture kept her completely out of action for three months. She said she couldn't believe how hard it was to accept her immobility. "It was like a grieving process; I couldn't stand to drive around the lakes and see other people running." As a result of that experience, Jean has diversified her sports and now pays careful attention to aches and pains that she feels may develop into more serious injuries.

In addition to dietary changes dictated by her diabetes, she and her family have also modified their eating habits over the years to cut out fat and salt. Recently, Jean also gave up caffeine after she realized that she was drinking eight to ten cups of coffee a day while writing her thesis. "Mainly I stopped because I didn't like the way it made me feel, and right now, I know moderation would be harder than quitting."

Because Jean has been physically active most of her life, and has always had a positive view of her body and what it can do, she says that the diabetes is sometimes difficult to accept. "All of a sudden it seems like I can't trust my body . . . the machine part of it is doing crazy and unpredictable things. Someone said maybe I should always run with someone . . . just in case. I see my independence linked to a body that works, or that I can rely on. I want to be in control." Jean says she is struggling to learn what changes she still needs to make so that she can be more sure of what to expect. Once she knows her limitations she is confident she can continue to do the things she loves to do.

Jean believes that taking care of herself is the number one priority. Without her own health, she knows it would be difficult to care for others. Putting herself first, however, does not necessarily come easily. In the last six months, Jean has made a conscious effort to nurture herself, part of which is to find a quiet time each day when she can "center." Running or other forms of exercise sometimes become the place for this quiet time, or it may be time that is spent reflecting or reading. She says balancing her work, parenting, relationships, and exercise is proving to be a continual challenge. Right now the balancing act is working, but Jean is keeping her eye on the scale, in case the demands of life threaten to tip the balance.

BETH, age sixty-seven

Today, Beth's favorite sports are walking and tennis. As a child she liked swimming, but "not competitive swimming," she says. "I just liked being in the water; it always made me feel comfortable." She also skated, played basketball, and tennis. Beth remembers starting to play golf at twelve or thirteen: "I always did a lot with my father, and I had an uncle who was always encouraging me to try new sports . . . it was because of him that I tried fencing and archery."

One of the only times Beth remembers being less than active was when her kids were young. She never entirely gave up tennis, however; she used to take the kids along in a stroller and park them on the sidelines while she played. Skating remained a special love and something that she continued to do until very recently. "Oh, not with figure skates, but hockey skates!" she says with a laugh.

Beth says that she never thought of walking as physical activity until recently. Now she tends to walk every day, not just leisurely walking, but at a good clip. "I amuse myself sometimes . . . when I know I am heading out for my walk, I start off down the hall of our condo at a much faster pace then normal!" Her lifelong commitment to tennis continues. She plays one and a half hours two times a week. One of the days she plays with a group of four women who have been getting together regularly for years. Having a structure makes the difference; knowing her tennis is planned at a regular time and with a regular group makes it a priority. Beth knows when she can't play it is her responsibility to get a "sub" and is glad that she knows many other women who can fill in. Beth also subs for another regular group of eight, and since many of these women and their spouses are near retirement and frequently out of town, she finds that she can play quite often. Both she and her spouse also play senior tennis, which has helped them meet a whole new set of acquaintances.

Beth has difficulty remembering anyone who discouraged her from being active; she credits the men in her life as being the most encouraging and supportive. She says her father, uncle, and spouse have all helped her try new things and keep active.

Competition is not a high priority for Beth. When she was in her late fifties and early sixties, she played on the "B" tennis team at a health club, but she has never been very enthusiastic about competing. "I've always played for fun," she says. Perhaps as a result, Beth has experienced no injuries; neither has she ever consciously altered other patterns such as eating or sleeping to improve performance.

Does exercise affect relationships? Beth recalls that her only time of really feeling depressed, discouraged, or trapped was when her children were little. Playing tennis and getting out helped relieve those emotions. Trying new forms of activity can also be a way of forming new relationships. Recently Beth has taken a yoga class through which she has started a few new friendships.

When asked if she has changed food preferences and habits over the years, Beth says, "Absolutely!" She thinks she is like "most intelligent people" who have greatly cut down on meat and solid fats. Beth also sees these "better" eating habits as a good way to control her weight while keeping her healthy.

Does being physically active change the way you perceive your body? Beth says she was convinced as a young child that posture was important, and feels that physical activity makes her stronger. She works at staying limber and takes pride in looking strong and active.

For Beth, feeding the emotional connections in her life is also an important part of taking care of herself. She sees many of her friends on a regular basis because they play tennis together. Her other social circles and her busy family life keep her lively and stimulated. Since Beth has always been part of an academic community, reading good books and having provocative discussions are all central to her sense of well-being. She belongs to several organizations that "require" members to do research and present papers. Walking, playing tennis, gardening, writing, and volunteering all make life in the late sixties very rich.

SARAH JANE, age sixty

Sarah Jane couldn't wait to turn sixty. Her birthday was the cause of much celebration because it meant a new race category and probably some new national age group records in running. Sarah Jane started running when she was fifty-four, and although her competitive success has made it her number one sport, she also loves to ride her bike and hike.

As a child Sarah Jane has few memories of any regular physical activity. She says she wanted a bike in the worst way, but that since it was the Depression she didn't get one until she was twelve. "It was my prized possession," she recalls. "I just loved it and rode it everywhere." The other physical activities Sarah remembers were unorganized and inexpensive—ice skating, sledding, and swimming.

In college Sarah Jane enjoyed dancing, but otherwise she was almost entirely inactive for fifteen years or more. She resumed biking in her mid-thirties and began seriously hiking five days a week. When her two children were in school she began swimming once a week at the Y with a friend. In 1977, her spouse heard a talk by George Sheehan that inspired him to begin running. For the next three Minnesota winters she sat by the TV and told him he was crazy when he returned with a frosted beard at the end of his three-mile run. "Finally," she said, "I decided that maybe I should try running, since it seemed to give him pleasure and make him feel better. But, I hated it! I got shin splints, my knees hurt, and my thighs hurt. I ran in tennis shoes for the first year." On her early outings her husband ran with her although his pace was much faster and his endurance much greater. After several weeks, as the aches and pains diminished, Sarah Jane's goal was to run three miles. It took her only three and a half months to achieve this goal. While some of her friends thought she was crazy, her family was very supportive.

No one, certainly not Sarah Jane, expected that she would be able to compete so successfully. Shortly after she reached her goal of running three miles she saw a woman in the grocery store who had just run in a ten-kilometer race. "I was astounded," says Sarah Jane. "I assumed you would be home lying on the couch after running that far!" Indeed Sarah Jane's first competition was noteworthy; she was sore for a month! Six months later she ran another race that was much more enjoyable, and by the end of the summer, she was winning her age division. Competition has become important; Sarah Jane is proud of her many trophies and age-group records. She goes to speed-work training once a week and tries to get more sleep before an especially big race. Most important, she loves the activity and the new friends she has met. She recently served as president of the local women's running club where her enthusiasm for running and life inspired many younger women to set new goals for themselves.

Sarah Jane usually runs six days a week at 5:45 A.M. A group of men and women started meeting casually at one of the lakes near her home and the pattern has become habitual. She likes that time of day and it is also the most convenient for her. "When I first ran, I frequently got out at 4:30 P.M., but that seemed to break up my day." Does someone who begins to run at age fifty-four, competes at distances including the marathon, and races almost every week get injured often? Surprisingly, Sarah Jane has been almost entirely injury-free. She thinks she is fairly sensible, has a good strong body, and has been lucky. She did break her wrist once in a freak bike accident, but even that didn't stop her from running for very long. During the first few days when the pain was bad, she walked in "nonrunning, heavy clothes and heavy shoes" so that she wouldn't be tempted to do a little slow running for a block or so. She ran as soon as the pain decreased, at first with a plaster cast, and then with a fiberglass cast that seemed to weigh almost nothing in comparison.

Sarah Jane thinks that exercise affects her relationships because it gives her such a feeling of good health. "I feel like my whole body is alive!" She doesn't see her life as stressful at this point, but thinks she could have used running as an outlet when her children were younger. "I'm sure I should have been running when they were teenagers!"

Even when she was not as physically active, Sarah Jane, who is a tall, strong-looking woman, was able to eat anything she wanted without worrying about her weight. Her friends are still envious of the large, nutritious meals she eats, and they tease her by claiming she chooses her races based on the refreshments they serve afterward. Although Sarah Jane doesn't diet per se, running has changed her family's food patterns somewhat. They were starting to make healthier food choices even before the running, however. She and her husband cut down on red meat years ago.

Sarah Jane says being physically active has definitely changed the way she perceives her body. "It's a great, functioning body," she says. "I'm very aware of that fact, and very thankful that I can do things most of my contemporaries can't." Taking care of herself is important to Sarah Jane. She feels that a good body, a good diet, and exercise are the ticket to living a quality life for a long time to come. To keep her mind as limber as her body, she plans to keep up with her active volunteer schedule. "Helping others fills me up," she says, "and lets me share some of the energy I am so thankful for."

MEGAN, age thirty-seven

Megan loves to ride horses and run. She also swims occasionally, because she likes "the feel of water on my body." As a young child, her only organized activity was gym class, and she remembers that the president's physical fitness test was a big event each year. She doesn't think she did very well! By age nine, she knew that her favorite physical activity was horseback riding.

In junior high, Megan attended a private school, and everyone in the small classes participated in physical activity. "There was a special sport per season and it was a great time." Switching to a large public high school marked the end of her sports days, and the beginning of inactivity. "My main sport during that period was boys," she says, laughing. She adds that only a few girls seemed to be active in sports, and these athletic girls were physically intimidating. The boys she was interested in did not think it was "cool" for a girl to be an athlete. Megan describes herself as mainly sedentary from ages twelve to twenty-four.

At age twenty-four, Megan decided that her lifestyle, which included heavy smoking, was unhealthy. "It's typical of my personality, she says, that I needed to do something drastic to stop. I chose running because I thought it was incompatible with smoking. I literally set out to redo my lifestyle!" Cheering from the sidelines was her older brother, Tom, who had always been a hero and example to her. He encouraged her to join him for his usual morning run at the Y. She loved to report her progress and recalls that Tom was the perfect support. "He didn't push, and he had the right manner. After several months running took on a life of its own; smoking and the need for encouragement were past history."

About two years later Megan decided to enter her first race. She found she could "shine." For the next three years competing became the focus of her running. "I was pretty intense, I raced every weekend, ran seventy miles a week, did speed work, and got injured." For a while this lifestyle was very satisfying, and she continued to get a lot of encouragement from her mother who even mapped out twenty-mile runs for Megan to try when she was home on visits. "She loved it while at the same time found it hard to believe that her 'unathletic' daughter was capable of racing; she leapt over a barrier to give me a huge hug when I finished the Boston Marathon!" When Megan began competing in the late 1970s, there were not many women on the road. While she sensed that a lot of people thought she was crazy, Megan recalls being proud and liking the feeling of being different.

A series of injuries convinced Megan that competition had become too important to her. It had become mentally difficult for her to handle any time off from running. She became depressed after her first injury and worried about losing her edge. She almost frantically found alternative exercises and put more time into her work. While she found that she hadn't lost much fitness, her hurry to return to high mileage and competition resulted in more frequent injuries. At the same time, she had reached a performance plateau; to take the next step and move from a thirty-nine minute ten-kilometer to something faster would take a major effort. Megan had to admit that it was time to redo her lifestyle again. She decided to cut back on her competition, and put higher priority on other things in her life.

Today, Megan is president of her own company and has rediscovered horseback riding. Two years ago, her interest was rekindled by a friend who casually asked her to go on a Sunday ride. Several months later she found the "perfect setting and arrangement" and realized just how much she had missed this sport. "I am a competitive person, and it wasn't too hard to talk me into competing, although I didn't really know what to expect." Megan finds the riding competition and training quite different from running; she has found a wonderful coach who gives her and her horse constant feedback so that improvement seems to be continual. "It's the relationship," she says, "the communication between me and my horse, that is so special. There's nothing I like better than being on a long ride where I feel that we are a beautiful, harmonious unit."

Does physical activity affect relationships? "Absolutely," replied Megan. She met her spouse because they both were runners and she finds that this bond remains strong. She cautions, however, that some sports, like riding, which take a substantial time commitment, can also create problems in a relationship. In order to fit in her riding, complete with an hour-long commute to the stables, Megan has curtailed her running and rearranged her work schedule so that the family time does not suffer.

Megan does not feel that these shifts in her physical activity or work schedule have hurt her relationships with friends, however. "I have a very small group of close friends," she reports. "I'm lucky that one is my business partner with whom I can discuss things on a daily basis if I desire. It may actually improve friendships," she says. "Learning to listen to my horse's needs has made me more sensitive and better able to listen to people."

Megan says the way she takes care of herself is to make "staying active" a priority. Her job situation, while demanding, is also one that affords flexibility. She sees a growing commitment to riding because it adds "such an incredible dimension to my life," making her more relaxed, easier to get along with, and happier than she has ever been.

PORTRAIT OF THE ACTIVE WOMAN

As these case histories suggest, there is no typical "active woman." Some of these women are married, some single or widowed; some have children and some do not. Their occupations include writing, teaching, counseling, owning a business, and volunteering. Several are full- or part-time students. Some women have always been physically active, whereas others began later in life. Two of these women have medical conditions that would make it easy to avoid physical activity, yet both report that exercise is central to their sense of health and well-being. For several of the women, physical activity is an important part of their self-definition. Others tell us that moderate exercise makes them feel better, but it may not always be a priority.

EARLY INFLUENCES

While the backgrounds of the women we interviewed are different, one common denominator is that most mid-life and older women had few opportunities to participate in organized sport when they were growing up. This lack of opportunity didn't stop them from finding outlets for their energies, however. The women fondly recalled their days of "running around," playing pick-up softball, and riding bikes "everywhere."

Good experiences with physical activity in the past laid the groundwork for future attitudes and behavior.

Parents were frequently credited with introducing these women to sport and encouraging physical activity. For women who did not have the support of their parents, making a decision to try sports on their own was more difficult. Most of the women we talked to said their fathers provided the most encouragement for their physical activity. This finding was reinforced by a Melpomene study of 430 masters runners (age forty plus) who said their fathers were far more encouraging than their mothers. One of the major reasons for this fatherly support may be the social context. The masters runners and many of the women we interviewed grew up during the period when their mothers were not very physically active. The Wilson report, which was commissioned by the Wilson Sporting Goods Company and the Women's Sports Foundation in 1987, had a similar finding with girls who were fifteen to eighteen. Forty-four percent said their father was the main source of encouragement.

Our current study with children makes us believe that this fatherly role is changing as more mothers become physically active themselves. Many adult women see the positive aspects of sport for the first time through their daughter's experiences and begin to offer important support. Many women regret that these opportunities did not exist when they were young and are anxious for their daughters to participate. In the same Wilson study cited above, young girls said their mother was the primary source of encouragement, with only 27 percent citing their father.

TEAM VERSUS INDIVIDUAL SPORTS

Women who did not have a sports background, particularly in team sports, are more likely to try an individual sport as an adult. Most of the women interviewed, for example, have selected physical activity, which can be done independently. Almost all of them say that they enjoy walking or hiking. Some prefer partner sports like tennis. Not only is the social context important but they also appreciate the extra incentive supplied by knowing someone else is counting on them to play.

In the past, team sports such as baseball, volleyball, and field hockey have not been available to adults in most communities. But this seems to be changing. Women's and coed softball for adults is growing rapidly across the country. Senior tennis leagues, open to men and women over age forty, offer free tennis lessons for those who have never played and provide opportunities for structured competition for those who are more skilled.

CHILDREN

Those who have had children note that the years when children were small was the period of time they were least active, but none of them completely abandoned exercise. "My one morning out included swimming at the Y with a friend," said both Sarah Jane and Emily. "I took the kids to the tennis court and let them play alongside," remembers Beth. For many of the women, childcare was their primary responsibility and few asked spouses to "babysit" so they could run or go for a walk. While there is much discussion of shared childcare in the media, women who participated in the Melpomene exercise and pregnancy studies in 1981 and 1983 continued to find that they had more difficulty scheduling exercise after the birth of their children.

FRIENDS

The importance of friends varies for these nine women. Some said that without friends they never would have started to exercise. Others said that friends are an added bonus but that they are not the real motivation to begin or to continue to exercise. For those who are married, however, some encouragement from a spouse made it more likely that they would exercise.

TIMING

Timing was important for all women interviewed. Some found that work schedules were the most important influence. The need to schedule around other aspects of busy lives was necessary for everyone; clearly physical activity must provide benefits or the effort will not be made. But it is also clear that there is no perfect time to exercise and that much depends on the time of day that "feels best" for the individual woman.

We hope that these interviews have inspired you to make your own decisions about an exercise plan that's right for you. There are no pat answers or prescriptions for fitness; each individual has her own unique approach to physical health. By painting a spectrum of possibilities, we hope you'll find a path that intrigues you.

* * *

Pierre de Coubertin, the originator of the modern Olympic games in 1896, said "Women's sports are against the laws of nature." In 1988, we watched an Olympic athlete named Florence Griffith Joyner beat a world record once set by the great Jesse Owens. As she streamed across the finish line, she hardly looked like she was defying the laws of nature. In fact, she looked as if nature had specially sculpted her for mercurial flight.

Despite what the skeptics would have us believe, physical activity is indeed part of a woman's nature. Our body is designed to perform beautifully—to swim, to run, to play, to grow strong, and to live vibrantly far into our older years. The vitality of young girls, teenagers, pregnant women, mid-life women, and seniors suggests that we are, by the laws of nature, built to live fully during all the phases of our lives.

When we exercise, our bodies change in ways that we are only just beginning to understand. Our lung power increases, our heart grows more robust, and we're better able to fight illnesses. Even our mind is quicker after a brisk walk. Perhaps the most important change, however, is what happens to our spirit as a result of vigorous play.

Again and again, women tell us that being in touch with their bodies puts them in touch with their abilities and with their inner promise. We hope that after reading this book, you will also feel more in tune with your body and better able to nurture and to challenge yourself. If you do, you'll be joining millions of other active women who, like the Greek Melpomene, are surprising the skeptics and turning the myths about active women inside out.

APPENDIX A

SOURCES OF INFORMATION
ABOUT
EATING DISORDERS

The following list may be helpful in gathering information about eating disorders:

The American Anorexia-Bulimia Association
  133 Cedar Lane
  Teaneck, NJ 07666
  Telephone: (201) 836-1800

ANAD-National Association of Anorexia Nervosa and Associated Disorders
  P.O. Box 7
  Highland Park, IL 60035
  Telephone: (312) 831-3438

ANRED-Anorexia Nervosa and Related Eating Disorders
  P.O. Box 5102
  Eugene, OR 97405
  Telephone: (503) 344-1144

Center for the Study of Anorexia Nervosa and Bulimia
  One West 91st Street
  New York, NY 10024
  Telephone: (212) 595-3449

National Anorexia Nervosa Aid Society
  5796 Karl Road
  Columbus, OH 43229
  Telephone: (614) 436-1112

BIBLIOGRAPHY

1: SHOULD "LADIES" BE ACTIVE?

Boutilier, Mary A., and SanGiovanni, Lucinda. 1983. *The Sporting Woman.* Champaign, IL: Human Kinetics Publishers.

Clarke, M. D., and Edward, H. 1873. *Sex in Education, or a Fair Chance for the Girls.* Boston: R. Osgood.

Drinkwater, Barbara L., ed. 1986. *Female Endurance Athletes.* Champaign, IL: Human Kinetics Publishers.

Dyer, K. F. 1982. *Challenging the Men: Women in Sport.* St. Lucia, Queensland, Australia: University of Queensland Press.

Ehrenreich, Barbara, and English, Dierdre. 1978. *For Her Own Good: 150 Years of the Experts' Advice to Women.* New York: Doubleday.

Gerber, Ellen W., Felshin, Jan, Berlin, Pearl, and Wyrick, Waneen. 1974. *The American Woman in Sport.* Philippines: Addison-Wesley Publishing Company.

Howe, Julia Ward, ed. 1874. *Sex and Education.* Boston: Roberts Bros.

Howell, Reet. 1982. *Her Story in Sport: A Historical Anthology of Women in Sports.* West Point, NY: Leisure Press.

Kaplan, Janice. 1979. *Women and Sports.* New York: Avon Books.

Metheney, Eleanor. 1965. *Connotations of Movement in Sport and Dance.* Dubuque, IA: Brown.

Miller Brewing Company. 1983. *The Miller Lite Report on American Attitudes Toward Sports.* Milwaukee, WI: Miller Brewing Company.

2: BODY IMAGE/BODY MIRAGE

Bailey, W. 1982. Women and their fat. *Covert Bailey Newsletter.* 2-3.

Bell, C., and Kirkpatrick, S. 1986. Body image of anorexic, obese, and normal females. *Journal of Clinical Psychology.* 42(3):431-439.

Bennet, N., and Gurin, J. 1982. The dieter's dilemma, in *Eating Less and Weighing More*. NY: Basic Books.

Brownell, K. 1982. Obesity: Understanding and treating a serious, prevalent and refractory disorder. *Journal of Consulting and Clinical Psychology*. 50(6):820-840.

Burk, J., Zelen, S., and Terino, E. 1985. More than skin deep: A self-consistency approach to the psychology of cosmetic surgery. *Plastic and Reconstructive Surgery*. 76(2):270-280.

Canning, H., and Mayer, J. 1966. Obesity—Its possible effect on college acceptance. *New England Journal of Medicine*. 245:1172-1174.

Connors, M., and Johnson, C. 1987. Epidemiology of bulimia and bulimic behaviors. *Addictive Behaviors*. 12:165-179.

Dahlkoetter, J., Callahan, E., and Linton, J. 1979. Obesity and the unbalanced energy equation: Exercise versus eating habit change. *Journal of Consulting and Clinical Psychology*. 47(5):898-905.

Dyrenforth, S., Wooley, O., and Wooley, S. 1980. A woman's body in a man's world: A review of findings on body image and weight control. In J. R. Kaplan (ed.), *A Woman's Conflict*. London: Prentice-Hall, pp. 31-57.

Eckholm, E. 1985. That lean and hungry look is no good as we age, controversial research says. *Saint Paul Pioneer-Press Dispatch*. August 25: IH, 6-7.

Eigner, J. 1986. Body image and self esteem. *Melpomene Report*. 8-12.

Fallon, A., and Rozin, P. 1985. Sex differences in perceptions of desirable body shape. *Journal of Abnormal Psychology*. 94(1):102-105.

Feldman, W., Feldman, E., and Goodman, J. T. 1988. Culture versus biology: Children's attitudes toward thinness and fatness. *Pediatrics*. 81(2):190-194.

Foster, C., Lutter, J., Denny, K., and Kimber, C. 1986. The Melpomene Institute body image study: A preliminary report. *Melpomene Report*. 5(1):3-8.

Freedman, R. 1984. Reflections on beauty as it relates to health in adolescent females. In S. Golub (ed.), *Health Care of the Female Adolescent*. NY: Haworth Press, pp. 29-45.

Garrow, J. S. 1974. *Energy Balance and Obesity in Man*. Amsterdam: North Holland.

Harris, M., and Smith, S. 1982. Beliefs about obesity: Effects of age, ethnicity, sex and weight. *Psychological Reports*. 51:1047-1055.

Haskew, P. 1985. Fat phobia: A cult that poses perils. *Medical Tribune*. 26:29.

Janelli, L. 1986. Body image in older adults: A review of the literature. *Rehabilitation Nursing*. 11(4):6-8.

Klesges, R., Mizes, J., and Kleges, L. 1987. Self-help dieting strategies in college males and females. *International Journal of Eating Disorders*. 6(3):409-417.

Lyons, P., and Ansfield, A. 1987. Body image and large women. *Melpomene Journal*. 7(1):6-9.

Lyons, P., and Burgard, D. 1988. *Great Shape: The First Exercise Guide for Large Women.* New York: Arbor House.

McBride, L. 1986. Teaching about body image: A technique for improving body satisfaction. *Journal of School Health.* 56(2):76-77.

Manson, J., Stampfer, M., Hennekens, C., and Willett, W. 1987. Body weight and longevity: A reassessment. *Journal of the American Medical Association.* 257(3):353-358.

Mendleson, B., and White, D. 1985. Development of self-body-esteem in overweight youngsters. *Developmental Psychology.* 21(1):90-96.

Monello, L., and Mayer, J. 1963. Obese adolescent girls: An unrecognized "minority" group? *American Journal of Clinical Nutrition.* 13:35-39.

Robinson, B. 1985. The stigma of obesity: Fat fallacies debunked. *Melpomene Report.* 4(1):9-13.

Robinson, J. 1983. Body image in women over forty. *Melpomene Report.* 2(3):12-14.

Storz, N., and Greene, W. 1983. Body weight, body image, and perception of fad diets in adolescent girls. *Journal of Nutrition Education.* 15(1):15-18.

Warviek, P., Toft, R., and Garrow, J. 1978. Individual differences in energy expenditure. In G. A. Gray (ed.), *Recent Advances in Obesity Research.* Vol. 2. London: Newman.

Wilson, T. 1987. Assessing treatment outcome in bulimia nervosa: A methodological note. *Internation Journal of Eating Disorders.* 6(3):339-348.

Zurek, L. 1987. Melpomene research update. *Melpomene Report.* 6(1):18.

3: MENSTRUAL FACT AND FICTION

Abraham, G. E. 1983. Nutritional factors in the etiology of premenstrual tension syndromes. *Journal of Reproductive Medicine.* 28(7):446-464.

Bell, M., and Parsons, E. 1930. Dysmenorrhea in college women. *Medical Women's Journal.* 38:31.

Benson, C. 1980. *Handbook of Obstetrics and Gynecology.* Los Altos, CA: Lange Medical Publications.

Bergfeld, J. A. et al. 1987. Women in athletics: Five management problems. *Patient Care.* 21(4), February 28.

Bergkvist, L., and Adami, H. O. et al. 1989. The risk of breast cancer after estrogen and estrogen-progestin replacement. *New England Journal of Medicine.* 321(5).

Brooks, S. M., and Sanborn, C. F. et al. 1984. Diet in athletic amenorrhea. *Lancet.* 559-560, March 10.

Brownell, K. D. and et al. 1987. Weight regulation practices in athletes: Analysis of metabolic and health effects. *Medicine & Science in Sports & Exercise.* 19(6):546-556.

Budoff, P. W. 1980. *No More Menstrual Cramps and Other Good News.* NY: G. P. Putnam & Sons.

Bullen, B. A. et al. 1985. Induction of menstrual disorders by strenuous exercise in untrained women. *New England Journal of Medicine.* 312:1349-1353.

Cann. C. E. et al. 1984. Decreased spinal mineral content in amenorrheic women. *Journal of American Medical Association.* 251(5):626-632, February 3.

Chauasse, P. H. 1888. *Wife and Mother, or, Information for Every Woman.* Philadelphia: H. J. Smith & Co.

Deuster, P. A. et al. 1986. Nutritional intakes and status of highly trained amenorrheic and eumenorrheic women runners. *Fertility and Sterility.* 46(4):636-643.

Drinkwater, B. L. et al. 1984. Bone mineral content of amenorrheic and eumenorrheic athletes. *New England Journal of Medicine.* 311:227-280.

Drinkwater, B. L. et al. 1986. Bone mineral density after resumption of menses in amenorrheic athletes. *Journal of the American Medical Association.* 256(3):380-382.

Fortino, D. 1987. Can exercise cure PMS? *Women's Sports and Fitness.* November: 311(5):44-47.

Frisch, R. E. et al. 1980. Delayed menarche and amenorrhea in ballet dancers. *New England Journal of Medicine.* 303(1).

Frisch, R. E., and McArthur, J. W. 1974. Menstrual cycles: Fatness as a determinant of minimum weight for height necessary for their maintenance of onset. *Science.* 185, September 13.

Frisch, R. E., and Revelle, R. 1970. Height and weight at menarche and a hypothesis of critical body weights and adolescent events. *Science.* 169:397-398.

Goldin, B. R. et al. 1982. Estrogen excretion patterns and plasma levels in vegetarian and omnivorous women. *New England Journal of Medicine.* 307:1542-1547.

Hensen, A. M., and Immordina, K. F. et al. 1984. The diagnostic evaluation and therapy of secondary amenorrhea. *Journal of Obstetrics and Gynological Nursing.* 13:180-184.

Jones, J. 1986. *P.M.S. Melpomene Report.* 5(1):12-17.

Lutter, J. M. 1983. Mixed messages about osteoporosis in female athletes. *Physician and Sportsmedicine.* 11(9).

Magyar, D. M., and Boyers, S. P. et al. 1979. Regular menstrual cycles and premenstrual molimina as indicators of ovulation. *Obstetrics and Gynecology.* 53(411).

Malina, R. et al. 1983. Menarche in athletes: A synthesis and hypothesis. *Annals of Human Biology.* 10(1):1-24.

Marcus, R. et al. 1985. Menstrual function and bone mass in elite women distance runners. *Annals of Internal Medicine.* 102:158-163.

Monahan, T. 1987. Treating athletic amenorrhea: A matter of instinct? *Physician and Sportsmedicine*. 15(7):184-189.

Nolen, J. 1965. Problems of menstruation. *Journal of Health, Physical Education and Recreation*. 36:65.

O'Brien, P. M. S. 1985. The premenstrual syndrome—a review. *Journal of Reproductive Medicine*. 30(2):113-125.

Prior, J. C. 1982. Endocrine "conditioning" with endurance training—a preliminary review. *Canadian Journal of Applied Sport Science*. 7(3):148-157.

Prior, J. C. 1985. Luteal phase defects and anovulation: Adaptive alterations occurring with conditioning exercise. In *Seminars in Reproductive Endrocrinology*. Vol. 3, series 1. Thieme-Stratton, Inc.

Prior, J. C. et al. 1987. Conditioning exercise decreases premenstrual symptoms: A prospective, controlled 6-month trial. *Fertility and Sterility*. 47(3):402-407.

Prior, J. C., and Vigna, Y. 1986. The therapy of reproductive system changes associated with exercise training. *The Menstrual Cycle and Physical Activity*. Champaign, IL: Human Kinetics Publishers.

Rebuffe-Scrive, M. et al. 1985. Fat cell metabolism in different regions in women. *Journal of Clinical Investigations*. 75:1973-1976.

Ruble, D. M., and Brooks-Gunn, J. 1979. Menstrual symptoms: A social condition analysis. *Journal of Behavioral Medicine*. 2(2):171-194.

Ryan, A. J. 1965. Gynecological considerations. *Journal of Health, Physical Education and Recreation*. 36:65.

Sanborn, C. F., Albrecht, B. H., and Wagner, W. W. 1987. Athletic amenorrhea: Lack of association with body fat. *Medicine and Science in Sport and Exercise*. 19(3):207-212.

Scott, E. D., and Johnson, F. E. 1982. Critical fat, menarche, and the maintenance of menstrual cycles. *Journal of Adolescent Health Care*. 2:249-260.

Shangold, M., and Mirkin, G. 1985. *The Complete Sports Medicine Book for Women*. NY: Simon & Schuster.

Ulrich, C. 1960. *Women and Sport-Science and Medicine of Exercise and Sports*. NY: Harper and Brothers.

Vancouver Women's Health Collective. 1985. *PMS: Premenstrual Syndrome, A Self-Help Approach*.

Warren, M. P. *Clinical Aspects of Menarche: Normal Variations and Common Disorders*. NY: College of Physicians and Surgeons, St. Luke's-Roosevelt Hospital. Columbia University.

Webb, J. L., Melan, D. L., and Stolz, C. J. 1979. Gynecological survey of American female athletes competing at Montreal Olympic Games. *Journal of Sports Medicine*. 19:405-412.

4: PREGNANCY AND FITNESS

Artal, R., and Wiswell, R. 1986. *Exercise in Pregnancy*. Baltimore, MD: Williams & Wilkins.

Berkowitz, G. S., Kelsey, J. L., Holford, T. R., and Berkwitz, R. L. 1983. Physical activity and the risk of spontaneous preterm delivery. *Journal of Reproductive Medicine*. 28(9):581-588.

Bolton, M. 1980. Scuba diving and fetal well-being. *Undersea Biomedical Research*. 7(3):183-189.

Briend, A. 1980. Maternal physical activity, birth weight and perinatal mortality. *Medical Hypotheses*. 6:556-562.

Chan, G. M., 1982. Human milk calcium and phosphate levels of mothers delivering term and pre-term infants. *Journal of Pediatrics, Gastroenterology and Nutrition*. 1:201-205.

Clapp, J., and Dickstein, S. 1984. Endurance exercise and pregnancy outcome. *Medicine and Science in Sports and Exercise*. 16(6):556-562.

Cohen, G. C., Prior, J. C., Vigna, Y., and Pride, S. M. Intense exercise during the first two trimesters of unapparent pregnancy. *Physician and Sportsmedicine*. 17(1):87-94, January 1989.

Collins, C., Curet, L., and Mullin J. 1983. Maternal and fetal response to a maternal aerobic exercise program. *Journal of Obstetrics and Gynecology*. 145(6):702-707.

Cox, J. 1987. Maternal nutrition during lactation. *ICEA Review*. 11(2):R1.

Danforth, D. 1967. Pregnancy and labor from the vantage point of the physical therapist. *Journal of Physical Medicine*. 46(1):653-658.

Dohrmann, K., and Lederman, S. A. 1986. Weight gain in pregnancy. *Journal of Obstetrical, Gynecological, and Neonatal Nursing*. Nov/Dec, 446-453.

Dressendorfer, R. H., and Goodlin, R. C. 1980. Fetal heart rate response to maternal exercise testing. *Physician and Sportsmedicine*. 8(11):91-94.

Erdelyi, G. 1962. Gynecological survey of female athletes. *Journal of Sports Medicine and Physical Fitness*. 12(3):174.

Erkkola, R. 1975. The physical fitness of Finnish primigravidae. *Annales Chirurgiae et Gynaecologiae Fenniae*. 64:394.

Exercise during pregnancy and the postnatal period. 1985. *American College of Obstetrics and Gynecology*. May.

Fast, V., Shapiro, D., Ducommun, E., and Friedmann, L. et al. 1987. Low back pain in pregnancy. *Spine*. 12(4):368-371.

Franz, M., Cooper, N., Mullen, L., and Bish, R. 1988. *Gestational Diabetes: Guidelines for a Safe Pregnancy and a Healthy Baby*. Wayzata, MN: International Diabetes Center.

Gauthier, M. 1986. Guidelines in exercise during pregnancy—too little or too much? *Physician and Sportsmedicine.* 14(4):162.

George, G., and Berk, B. 1981. Exercise before, during and after pregnancy. *Topics in Clinical Nursing.* 3(2):33-39, July.

Gestational Diabetes: Guidelines for a Safe Pregnancy and a Healthy Baby. 1988. International Diabetes Center, Wayzata, MN.

Gorski, J. 1985. Exercise during pregnancy: Maternal and fetal responses: A brief review. *Medicine and Science in Sports and Exercise.* 17(4):407-416.

Guzman, C. A., and Caplan, R. 1970. Cardiorespiratory response to exercise during pregnancy. *American Journal of Obstetrics and Gynecology.* 108:600.

Hall, D., and Kaufmann, D. 1987. Effects of aerobic and strength conditioning on pregnancy outcome. *American Journal of Obstetrics and Gynecology.* 157(5):1199-1203.

Hon, H. H., and Wohlgemuth, R. 1961. The electronic evaluation of fetal heart rate. *American Journal of Obstetrics and Gynecology.* 81(2):361.

Hong, S. K., and Rahn, H. 1967. The diving women of Korea and Japan. *Scientific American.* 216(5):34-43.

Hutchinson, P., Cureton, K. J., and Sparling, P. B. 1981. Metabolic and circulatory responses to running during pregnancy outcome. *Physician and Sportsmedicine.* 9(8):55.

Jarrett, J., and Spellacy, W. 1983. Jogging during pregnancy: An improved outcome? *Obstetrics and Gynecology.* 61:705.

Jones, R., Botti, J., Anderson, W., and Bennett, N. 1985. Thermoregulation during aerobic exercise in pregnancy. *Obstetrics and Gynecology.* 65(3):340-345.

Jovanovic, L., Kessler, A., and Peterson, C. 1985. Human maternal and fetal responses to graded exercise. *Journal of Applied Physiology.* 58(5):1719-1722.

Jutel, A. 1986. Running while pregnant. *Washington Running Report*, March/April, 8-9.

Kizer, K. 1980. Medical hazards of the water skiing douche. *Annals of Emergency Medicine.* 9(5):268.

Kizer, K. 1983. Women and diving. *Physician and Sportsmedicine.* 9(2):85.

Kris-Etherton, P. M. 1986. Nutrition and the exercising female. *Nutrition Today.* March/April, 21(2):6-18.

Kulpa, P., White, B., and Visschler, R. 1987. Aerobic exercise in pregnancy. *American Journal of Obstetrics and Gynecology.* 156(6):1395-1403.

Ledermann, S. 1985. Physiological changes of pregnancy and the relationship to nutrient needs. *Current Concepts in Nutrition.* 14:12-43.

Lee, V., and Lutter, J. 1988. Exercise and pregnancy: Choices, concerns, and recommendations. In E. Wilder (ed.), *Obstetric and Gynecologic Physical Therapy.* NY: Churchill Livingstone, 175-198.

Lotgering, F., Gilbert, R., and Longo, L. 1984. Interactions of exercise and pregnancy: A review. *American Journal of Obstetrics and Gynecology.* 149(5):560-568.

Lotgering, F., and Longo, L. 1984. Exercise and pregnancy—how much is too much? *Contemporary Obstetrics and Gynecology.* January. 63-77.

McMurray, R. G., Katz, V. L., and Goodwin, W. 1988. Pregnancy, thermoregulation and exercise in water. Paper presented at ACSM, May 25.

Maternal physical activity effects on the fetus and pregnancy outcome, 1976. *International Childbirth Education Association Review.* 10(1):1-8.

Morris, N. et al. 1956. Effective uterine bloodflow during exercise in normal and pre-eclamptic pregnancies. *Lancet.* 2, 481-484.

Mullinax, K., and Dale, E. 1986. Some considerations of exercise and pregnancy. *Clinics in Sports Medicine.* 5(3):559-570.

Paolone, A., Shangold, M., and Paul, D. et al. 1987. Fetal heart rate measurement during maternal exercise—avoidance of artifact. *Medicine and Science in Sports and Exercise.* 19(6):605-609.

Pirie, L. B., and Curtis, L. R. 1987. *Pregnancy and Sports Fitness.* Tucson, AZ: Fisher Books.

Pleet, H., and Graham, J. et al. 1981. Central nervous system and facial defects associated with maternal hypothermia at four to fourteen weeks' gestation. *Pediatrics.* 67:785.

Polden, A. 1985. Teaching postnatal exercise. *Midwives Clinical and Nursing Notes.* October, 271-274.

Pomerance, J. J., Gluck, L., and Lynch, V. 1983. Physical fitness in pregnancy, its effect on pregnancy outcome. *American Journal of Obstetrics and Gynecology.* 119(9):867.

Regnier, S. 1987. *Exercises for Baby and Me.* NY: Meadowbrook.

Richards, D. 1985. Guidelines for exercise during pregnancy. *Occupational Health Nursing.* 33(10):508-509.

Ruhling, R. O., Cameron, J., and Sibley, L. et al. 1981. Maintaining aerobic fitness while jogging through a pregnancy: A case study. *Medicine and Science in Sports and Exercise.* 13(2):93.

Sady, S. P., Carpenter, M. W., and Sady, M. A. et al. 1988. Predication of VO2 Max. in pregnant women. *Journal of Applied Physiology.* 65:(2).

Sady, S. P., Carpenter, M. W., and Thompson, P. D. et al. 1989. The cardiovascular response to cycle exercise during and after pregnancy. *Journal of Applied Physiology.* 66(1):336-341.

Sherry, E. 1985. Pregnancy as a risk factor for injury in downhill skiing. *Medical Journal of Australia.* 143:633.

Sibley, L. 1981. Swimming and physical fitness during pregnancy. *Journal of Nurse Midwifery.* 26(6):3.

Slavin, J., Lutter, J. M., Cushman, S., and Lee, V. 1985. Pregnancy and exercise. *Sport Science Perspective for Women.* Proceedings from USOC Conference, Colorado Springs, Nov. 1985.

Speroff, L. 1980. Can exercise cause problems in pregnancy and menstruation? *Contemporary Obstetrics and Gynecology* 15:57-70.

Shangold, M., and Mirkin, G. 1985. *The Complete Sportsmedicine Book for Women.* NY: Simon & Schuster.

Uhari, M., and Mustonen, A. 1979. Sauna habits of Finnish women during pregnancy. *British Medical Journal.* 1:1216.

Veille, J. C., and Hohimer, A. R. et al. 1985. Effect of exercise on uterine activity in the last eight weeks of pregnancy. *American Journal of Obstetrics and Gynecology.* 151(6):727-730.

Wallace, A. M., and Engstrom, J. L. 1987. Effects of aerobic exercise on the pregnant woman, fetus and pregnancy outcome. *Journal of Nurse Midwifery.* 32(5):277-290.

Wardlaw, G., and Pike, A. 1986. Effect of lactation on peak adult shaft and ultra-distal forearm bone mass in women. *American Journal of Clinical Nutrition.* 44:283-286.

Wong, S. C., and McKenzie, D. C. 1987. Cardiorespiratory fitness during pregnancy and its effect on outcome. *International Journal of Sport Medicine.* 8:79-83.

Worthington-Roberts, B. 1984. Nutrition and maternal health. *Nutrition Today.* November/December.

Worthington-Roberts, B., Vermeersch, J., and Williams, S. 1985. *Nutrition in Pregnancy and Lactation.* St. Louis: Times Mirror/Mosby.

Zaharieva, E. 1972. Olympic participation by women: Effects on pregnancy and childbirth. *Journal of the American Medical Association.* 221(9):992.

5: RAISING YOUR CHILD TO BE ACTIVE

Andres, F., Rees, C.R., Weiner, S., and Weiss, D. 1981. Actual and perceived strength differences. *Journal of Physical Education, Recreation, and Dance.* 52:20-21.

Anthrop, J., and Allison, M. T. 1983. Role conflict and the high school female athlete. *Research Quarterly for Exercise and Sport.* 54:1040-1111.

Auchincloss, E. 1989. Sports: A field of opportunity for girls. *Melpomene Journal.* 8(1):8-10.

Bird, A. M., and Williams, J. M. 1980. A developmental-attributional analysis of sex-role stereotypes in sport performance. *Developmental Psychology.* 16:319-322.

Boutilier, Mary A., and SanGiovanni, L. (eds.). 1983. *The Sporting Woman.* Champaign, IL: Human Kinetics Publishers, Inc.

Coakley, J. 1980. Play, games and sport: Developmental implications for young people. *Journal of Sport Behavior*. 3:99-118.

Corbin, C., and Nix, C. 1979. Sex typing of physical activities and success predictions for children before and after cross-sex competition. *Journal of Sport Psychology*. 1:43-52.

Chapman, E., and Jones, C., 1988. Teenage Athletes: Striving for Personal Bests. *Melpomene Journal*. 7(2):11-13.

Corbin, Charles B. 1987. Youth fitness, exercise and health: there is much to be done. *Research Quarterly for Exercise and Sport*. December, 54(4).

Douctre, G. P., and Harris, G. A. 1983. An analysis of the self-image differences of male and female athletes. *Journal of Sport Behavior*. 6:77-83.

Duquin, M. E. 1978. The androgynous advantage. In C. A. Oglesby (ed.), *Women and Sport: From Myth to Reality*. Philadelphia: Lea & Febiger.

Fein, G., Johnson, D., Kosson, N., Stork, L., and Wasserman, L. 1975. Sex stereotypes and preferences in the toy choices of 20-month-old boys and girls. *Development Psychology*. 11:527-528.

Foster, C. D. 1983. Learning to deal with success and failure: Children's causal attributions. *Melpomene Report*. 2:11-13, May.

Gabbard, Carl P., and Crouse, S. 1988. Children and exercise: Myth and facts. *The Physical Educator*. Winter, 45(1).

Gilliam, T. B., Katch, V. et al. 1977. Prevalence of coronary heart disease risk factors in active children, 7 to 12 years of age. *Medicine and Science in Sports*. Vol. 9, 21-25.

Gilbert, S. 1978. *Feeling Good: A Book About You and Your Body*. NY: Four Winds Press.

Goldberg, S., and Lewis M. 1969. Play behavior in the year-old infant: Early sex differences. *Child Development*. 40:21-31.

Hall, E. G., and Lee, A. M. 1981. Sex and birth order in children's goal setting and actual performance of a motor task. *Perceptual and Motor Skills*. 53:663-666, October.

Hall, M. A. 1978. *Sport and Gender: A Feminist Perspective on the Sociology of Sport*. Vanier City, Ottowa, Ont: Canadian Association for Health, Physical Education, and Recreation.

Hoferek, M. J. 1982. Sex-role prescriptions and attitudes of physical educators. *Sex Roles*. 8:83-98.

Holland, M. 1988. Fitness for kids: An approach that works. *Melpomene Journal*. 7(3):22.

Knouse, S. B. 1982. Male and female stereotypes of game-playing abilities. *Perceptual and Motor Skills*. 55:543-545.

Kolata, G. 1986. Obese children: A growing problem. *Science*. April.

Lauer, R. M., Connor, W. E., and Leaverton, P. E. 1975. Coronary heart disease risk factors in school children muscatine study. *Journal of Pediatrics*. 86:697-706.

McHugh, M., Duquin, M., and Freize, I. 1978. Beliefs about success and failure: Attribution and the athlete. In C. Oglesby (ed.), *Women and Sport: From Myth to Reality.* Philadelphia: Lea & Febiger.

Montemayor, R. 1974. Children's performance in a game and their attraction to it as a function of sex-typed labels. *Child Development.* 45:152-156.

Montoye, H. J. 1985. Physical activity, physical fitness and heart disease risk factors in children. In G. Alan Stull and Helen Eckert (eds.), Effects of physical activity on children. *American Academy of Physical Education Papers.* No. 19, 57th annual meeting, April 15-16, Human Kinetics Publications.

Morris, A. M., Williams, J. M., Atwater, A. E., and Wilmore, J. H. 1983. Age and sex differences in motor performance of three 6-year-old children. *Research Quarterly.* 53:214-221.

National Center for Health Statistics, January 1974. *Preliminary Findings of First Health, Nutrition Examination Survey.* U.S., 1971-1972.

Novak Johnson, V. 1987. Children's sports socialization study. *Melpomene Journal.* 6(1):15-17.

Novak Johnson, V. 1988. Children's socialization into sport study. *Melpomene Journal.* 7(1):13.

Novak Johnson, V. 1988. Melpomene research reports: Children's socialization into sport study. *Melpomene Journal.* 7(2):15-20.

Pate, R. R., and Ross, J. G. 1987. The national children and youth fitness study II: Factors associated with health-related fitness. *Journal of Physical Education, Recreation and Dance.* November/December, 45-48.

Pollis, N., and Doyle, D. 1972. Sex role, status, and perceived competence among first graders. *Perceptual and Motor Skills.* 34:235-238.

Pogrebin, L. C. 1980. *Growing Up Free: Raising Your Child in the 80s.* NY: McGraw-Hill Book Co.

Pogrebin, L. C. 1982. *Stories for Free Children.* NY: McGraw-Hill Book Co.

Rajeski, W. 1980. Causal attribution: An aid to understanding and motivation. *Motor Skills: Theory into Practice.* 4:32-36.

Rajeski, W., and Brawley, L. 1983. Attribution theory in sport: Current status and new perspectives. *Journal of Sport Psychology.* 3:206-216.

Reiff, G. 1986. The President's council on physical fitness and sports: 1985 national school population fitness survey. Washington D.C., President's Council on Physical Fitness and Sports.

Ross, J. G., and Gilbert. 1985. The national children and youth fitness study: A summary of findings. *Journal of Physical Education, Recreation and Dance.* November/December.

Ross, J. G., and Pate, R. R. 1987. The national children and youth fitness study

II: A summary of findings. *Journal of Physical Education, Recreation and Dance.* November/December.

Shapiro, J. E. 1982. Locus of control: A neglected measure for affective development in physical education. *Physical Educator.* 39:126-130.

Sherif, C. W., and Rattray, G. 1976. Psychosocial development and activity in middle childhood: 5 to 12 years. In J. G. Albinson and G. M. Andrew (eds.), *Child in Sport and Physical Activity.* Baltimore: University Park Press.

Shipard, R., quoted in Londer, R., June 1987. Lazy bones, lagging bodies: Shaping up the next generation. *Child.* 48-49.

Snyder, E. E., and Spreitzer, E. 1976. Correlates of sport participation among adolescent girls. *Research Quarterly.* 47:804-809.

Strong, W. B., and Wilmore, J. H. 1988. "Unfit kids: An office-based approach to physical fitness," *Contemporary Pediatrics.* April.

Thatcher, J., quoted in Weaver, S. 1987. Turning kids on to fitness. *Children.* 55-56.

Wilcox, R. C. 1988. Promoting parents as partners in physical education. *The Physical Educator.* Winter, 45(1).

Wilson Sporting Goods Company, and the Women's Sports Foundation. 1988. Moms, dads, daughters, and sports. *The Wilson Report.* June 7.

6: AGE AND THE ACTIVE WOMAN

Abelson, D. J. 1986. The osteoporotic syndrome. *The Bulletin.* 30(1).

Adams, R. G. 1987. Patterns of network change: A longitudinal study of friendships of elderly women. *Gerontologist.* 27(2).

American Association of Retired Persons. 1986. *A Profile of Older Americans.* Program Resources Dept.

Bergkvist, L., and Adami, H. O. et al. 1989. The risk of breast cancer after estrogen and estrogen-progestin replacement. *New England Journal of Medicine.* Vol. 321, No. 5.

Block, J. E., and Smith, R. 1987. Overview of exercise and bone mass. In Harry K. Genant (ed.), *Osteoporosis Update 1987.* San Francisco: Radiology Research and Education Foundation.

Brodigan, D. E. 1989. *Melpomene Journal.* 8(1):22-23.

Clark, B. A. 1985. Principles of physical activity programming for the older adult. *Topics in Geriatric Rehabilitation.* 1(1):68.

Cook, J. 1986. Stop brittle bones. *Self.* December. 114-119.

Cummings, S. R. 1987. Epidemiology of osteoporotic fractures. In Harry K. Genant (ed.), *Osteoporosis Update 1987.* San Francisco: Radiology Research and Education Foundation.

Cummings, S. R. 1987. Use of bone density measurements. In Harry K. Genant (ed.), *Osteoporosis Update 1987*. San Francisco: Radiology Research and Education Foundation.

Cummings, S. R., and Black, D. B. 1986. Should perimenopausal women be screened for osteoporosis? *Annual of Internal Medicine*. 104:817.

Diokno, A. C., Wells, T. J., and Brink, C. A. 1987. Urinary incontinence in elderly women: Urodynamic evaluation. *Journal of the American Geriatric Society*. 35:940-946.

Doress, P. B., and Siegal, D. L. 1987. *Ourselves, Growing Older*. NY: Simon & Schuster.

Dorfman, L. T., and Moffett, M. M. 1987. Retirement satisfaction in married and widowed rural women. *Gerontologist*. 27(2):215.

Edwards, P. 1985. Keep your bones healthy. *Canadian Living*. 192-196.

Ettinger, B. 1987. Estrogen, progestogen, and calcium in treatment of postmenopausal women. In Harry K. Genant (ed.), *Osteoporosis Update 1987*. San Francisco: Radiology Research and Education Foundation.

Gambrell, D. R. 1986. Safety of estrogen-progestone replacement. 71-80. *Postgraduate Medicine*.

Gass, K. A. Coping strategies of widows. 1987. *Journal of Gerontological Nursing*. 13(8):29.

Hammond, M. G. 1984. The menopausal years: What to expect. *Drug Therapy*. December.

Harris, H., and Harris, S. 1989. *Physical Activity, Aging and Sports, Vol. 1, Scientific and Medical Research*. Albany, NY.

Harris, R., and Frankel, L. J. 1977. *Guide to Fitness After 50*. NY: Plenum Press.

Heaney, R. P. 1988. Dietary calcium and osteoporosis. *Nutrient*. 1(1).

Heaney, R., and Barger-Lux, M. 1988. *Calcium and Common Sense*. NY: Doubleday.

Hedlund, L. R., and Gallagher, J. C. 1988. Estrogen therapy for postmenopausal osteoporosis: Current status. *Geriatric Medicine Today*. 7(2):55-64.

Hurley, O. 1988. *Safe Therapeutic Exercise for the Frail Elderly: An Introduction*. NY: The Center for the Study of Aging.

Keith, P. M. 1987. Postponement of health care by unmarried older women. *Women & Health*. 12(1):47.

Kirkpatrick, M. K., and Edwards, K. 1985. Osteoporosis: A self-care check list for women. *Occupational Health Nursing*. 33:500.

Lutter, J. M. 1983. Bone mass loss and the athletic lifestyle. *Melpomene Report*. 2(1):7-8.

Lutter, J. M., Merrick, S., Steffen. L., Jones, C., and Slavin, J. 1985. Physical activity through the life span: Long-term effects of an active lifestyle. *Melpomene Report*. 4(1):15-18.

McElmurry, B. J., and LiBrizzi, S. J. 1986. The health of older women. *Nursing Clinics of North America*. 21(1):161.

Mattson, A. 1984. Controlling osteoporosis with exercise, diet and hormone therapy. *Melpomene Report*. 3(1):3-6.

Neimark, J. 1986. Beyond calcium: Why milk is just a start. *American Health*. October.

Niewoehner, C. 1987. Osteoporosis—Ongoing questions. Presentation of Continuing Medical Education, University of Minnesota.

Notelovitz, M., and Ware, M. 1982. *Stand Tall! The Informed Woman's Guide to Preventing Osteoporosis*. Gainesville, FL: Triad Publishing Co.

Riddick, C. C. 1985. Life satisfaction for older female homemakers, retirees, and workers. *Research on Aging*. 7(3):383.

Riggs, L., and Melton, L. J. 1986. Involutional osteoporosis. *New England Journal of Medicine*. 314(26):1676.

Samuels, M., and Zina Bennett, H. 1983. *Well Body, Well Earth*. San Francisco: Sierra Club Books.

Shannon, M. D. 1984. *Long Term Care of the Aging*. NJ: Slack Inc.

Shephard, R. J. 1986. Physiological aspects of sport and physical activity in the middle and later years of life. In Barry D. McPherson (ed.), *Sport and Aging*. Champaign, IL: Human Kinetics Publications, Inc.

Slavin, J. L. 1984. Nutrient intakes of osteoporosis study participants. *Melpomene Report*. 3(3):13-15.

Smith, E. L. 1982. Exercise for prevention of osteoporosis: A review. *Physician and Sportsmedicine*. 10(3):72.

Smith, E. L., and Gilligan, C. 1983. Physical activity prescription for the older adult. *Physician and Sportsmedicine*. 11:91-101.

Stoedefalke, K. G. 1985. Motivating and sustaining the older adult in an exercise program. *Topics in Geriatric Rehabilitation*. 1(1):78.

Voda, A. 1981. Alterations of the menstrual cycle. *The Menstrual Cycle, Vol. II* Ed. P. Komnenich. NY: Springer Publishing.

Voda, A. M. 1982. Coping with the menopausal hot flash. *Patient Counsel, Health Education*. 2:80-83.

Voda, A. 1984. *Menopause, Me and You*. Salt Lake City, UT: University of Utah.

Wilson, R. A. 1966. *Feminine Forever*. NY: M. Evans Press.

Zurek, E. M. 1987. Osteoporosis study update. *Melpomene Report*. Winter.

7: CHOOSING AN ACTIVE LIFESTYLE

Albohm, M. 1981. *Health Care and the Female Athlete*. North Palm Beach, FL: The Athletic Institute.

Anderson, B. 1980. *Stretching*. Bolinas, CA: Shelter Publications.

Calhoun, D. W. 1987. *Sport, Culture, and Personality*, 2nd ed. Champaign, IL: Human Kinetics Publishers.

Darden, E. 1983. *Especially for Women*. NY: Leisure Press.

Fait, H., and Dunn, J. 1984. *Special Physical Education: Adapted, Individualized, Developmental*, 5th ed. Dubuque, IA: William C. Brown Publishers.

Glover, B., and Shepherd, J. 1989. *The Family Fitness Handbook*. NY: Penguin Books.

Golding, L. A., Myers, C. R., and Sinning, W. 1989. *Y's Way to Physical Fitness*, 3rd ed. Champaign, IL: Leisure Press.

Harris, D., and Harris, B. 1984. *The Athlete's Guide to Sports Psychology: Mental Skills for Physical People*. NY: Leisure Press.

Ralston, J. 1986. *Walking for the Health of It*. Washington, DC: AARP.

Ritter, M. A., and Albohm, M. J. 1987. *Your Injury*. Indianapolis, IN: Benchmark Press.

Rotella, R. J., and Bunker, L. K. 1987. *Parenting Your Superstar*. Champaign, IL: Leisure Press.

Sharkey, B. J. 1984. *Physiology of Fitness*, 2nd ed. Champaign, IL: Leisure Press.

Ullyot, J. 1980. *Running Free*. NY: G. P. Putnam's Sons.

Wilmore, J. H. 1986. *Sensible Fitness*, 2nd ed. Champaign, IL: Leisure Press.

INDEX

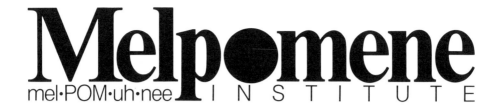

For Women's Health Research

Founded in 1981, Melpomene Institute identifies and researches health issues important to physically active women. Access to this information is provided through our Resource Center, information packets, brochures, and talks. We also present educational programs and conferences.

Join us!

We answer important questions about women's health and physical activity. A thirty-two dollar membership includes these benefits:

- Subscription to the Melpomene Journal, which contains the most current information on a variety of women's health topics.
- Resources, including article reprints, bibliographies, books, and videotapes.
- Discounts on conference fees, video rentals, literature searches, annual special events, talks arranged through Melpomene's speakers bureau.

Please send me more information about:

☐ Membership in Melpomene
☐ Melpomene speakers bureau
☐ Melpomene Resource Center
☐ Participation in a research study

Name _____

Address _____

City _____ State _____ Zip _____

Phone (work) _____ (home) _____

Please clip and mail to Melpomene Institute, 1010 University Avenue, St. Paul, MN 55104.